Harald Becher · Peter N Burns
Handbook of Contrast Echocardiography
Left ventricular function and myocardial perfusion

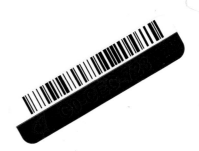

Springer
*Berlin
Heidelberg
New York
Barcelona
Hongkong
London
Milan
Paris
Singapore
Tokyo*

Harald Becher · Peter N Burns

Handbook of Contrast Echocardiography
Left ventricular function and myocardial perfusion

With a foreword by

Sanjiv Kaul, MD
Professor of Cardiology
Director of Cardiovascular Imaging Center
University of Virginia

Impressum

Peter N Burns
Professor of Medical Biophysics and Radiology
University of Toronto
Imaging Research
Sunnybrook and Women's Health Science Centre
2075 Bayview Avenue
Toronto, Ontario
Canada M4N 3M5

Harald Becher
Professor of Cardiology
University of Bonn
Rheinische Friedrich-Wilhelms-Universität
Medizinische Universitätsklink und Poliklink II
Kardiologie/Pneumologie
Sigmund-Freud-Straße 25
53105 Bonn
Germany

ISBN 3-540-67083-1 Springer-Verlag Berlin Heidelberg New York

---

Library of Congress Cataloging-in-Publication Data
Becher, Harald
Handbook of Contrast Echocardiography: LV Function and Myocardial Perfusion
/Harald Becher and Peter N Burns p.cm.
Includes bibliographical references and index.
ISBN 3540670831 (alk. paper)
1. Ultrasonic cardiography - Handbooks, manuals, etc.
2. Heart - Diseases - Diagnosis - Handbooks - manuals, etc. I. Burns,
Peter N. II. Title
RC683.5.U5 B43 2000   616.1'207543--dc21
                                 00-026586

Copyright © 2000 by Harald Becher and Peter N Burns. All rights reserved. This book is protected by copyright. No part of it may be reproduced, stored in a retrieval system, or transmitted, in any form or by any means, electronic, mechanical, photocopying, recording, or otherwise, without prior written permission of the copyright owners.

This work is subject to copyright. All rights are reserved, whether the whole part of material is concerned, specifically the rights of translation, reprinting, reuse of illustrations, recitation, broadcasting, reproduction on microfilm.

The use of general descriptive names, registerd names, trademarks, etc. in this publication does not imply, even in the absence of a specific statement, that such names are exempt from the relevant protective laws and regulations and therefore free for general use.

Set and Production by Bengelsdorf & Schimmel, Gesellschaft für visuelle Kommunikation mbH, Berlin
Printed by Druckcentrum Fürst, Berlin

Foreword

Although the technology required for the successful application of contrast echocardiography has evolved rapidly over the past few years, the technique has not yet gained widespread clinical acceptance. One important reason for the lack of clinical acceptance is the relative complexity of the technique, particularly in respect to myocardial perfusion imaging. The interaction between microbubbles and ultrasound is an entire field by itself, as is the coronary microvasculature.

It is in this regard that practicing echocardiographers, cardiologists in training, radiologists, sonographers, and students will find 'A Handbook of Contrast Echocardiography' particularly useful. Written by two leaders in the field who have presented illustrative cases not only from their own laboratories but also from others around the world, this volume is a lucid, concise, and practical guide for the day-to-day use of contrast echocardiography.

Dr Peter Burns has been involved in almost all the technical advances in the imaging methods that have made it possible to detect opacification of the left ventricular cavity and myocardium from a venous injection of microbubbles. He has been responsible to a large degree for advancing our understanding of the interaction between microbubbles and ultrasound, which he describes in clear and easy to understand terms in this book. Dr Harald Becher has been active in the clincal application of contrast echocardiography for several years and has gained considerable experience with many imaging techniques and microbubbles, which he describes in this volume in some detail.

The reader will find 'A Handbook of Contrast Echocardiography' very useful to get them started in contrast echocardiography. The answer to almost any question that may come up in the initial period of one's training in this method will be found in this book. The authors and publishers should be congratulated for making available a very useful and welcome addition to the armamentarium required to make one a successful practitioner in the art and science of contrast echocardiography.

Sanjiv Kaul, MD

Charlottesville, Virginia, USA
April, 2000

Preface

The injection of a contrast agent forms a routine part of clinical x-ray, CT, MR and radionuclide imaging of the heart and vascular system. Yet in spite of the obvious significance of the vascular component of the echocardiographic examination, and in spite of widespread experimentation with contrast agents for ultrasound, ultrasound imaging of the heart has only just begun to exploit the potential benefit of contrast enhancement. Why?

A typical response from echocardiographers new to contrast is that intravascular injections would detract from one of ultrasound's major attractions, that it is noninvasive. Yet, if it can be shown that the additional diagnostic information obtained with contrast enhancement will spare the patient from a more invasive procedure, it would be doing them no favour to deny them a painless venous injection. A more fundamental consideration appeals to the nature of the ultrasound image itself, which benefits from an intrinsically high contrast between blood and solid tissue. It could be argued that, unlike x-ray angiography, ultrasound does not need a contrast agent and an associated subtraction imaging method to 'see' blood. If we are interested in visualising where the blood flows, colour Doppler imaging offers a powerful and effective tool, providing the additional ability to quantify hemodynamic parameters such as the direction and velocity of flow.

In the early days of echocardiography, a B-mode image could depict the cavity of a cardiac chamber but not whether blood was flowing across a septal defect. Free gas bubbles were injected into the cavity and their trajectory imaged: this was really the first use of a contrast agent in ultrasound. Yet this invasive procedure, which requires catheterisation, is often no longer necessary. Colour Doppler imaging has largely supplanted the intra-arterial injection of bubbles in cardiac diagnosis and its capabilities now define the flow information obtainable in echocardiography.

It is precisely these capabilities that the new generation of ultrasound contrast agents for cardiac diagnosis has extended, redefining the role of echocardiography and acting at all levels of the examination. In imaging modes, contrast agents can help delineate the endocardial border, improving the success rate of wall motion studies. In Doppler modes, the agents boost the echo from blood, allowing detection of epicardial vessels that would otherwise fail. Finally, and most exciting of all, the agents make it possible for ultrasound to achieve entirely new objectives, the most striking of which is the ability for the first time to image perfusion of the myocardium in real time. This books aims to provide both a guide and a reference for the practical use of contrast agents for these new indications.

In Chapter 1, the fundamental principle of contrast enhancement for echocardiography is described and the mode of action of currently available microbubble agents explained. The various imaging methods that have been developed to make their use more effective are discussed along with guidelines for their clinical application. Chapter 2 addresses the use of contrast echocardiography in assessing left ventricular function. The specific indications for contrast are proposed and its role set in the context of other clinical examinations of systolic and diastolic function. Practical, step-by-step instructions are given for using contrast in Doppler, wall motion and ejection fraction studies and their incorporation into the stress echo examination.

Chapter 3 is devoted to imaging blood perfusion at the tissue level with ultrasound, the newest and most demanding application of contrast. The physiology and pathophysiology of myocardial perfusion are reviewed and the role of the echo examination discussed. Protocols are provided for the new techniques of harmonic imaging, harmonic power angio, pulse inversion and power pulse inversion and the use of the different agents explained. Although these technologies are evolving rapidly, current recommendations for specific instrument settings are included for each examination, with a careful explanation of their significance together with guidelines for keeping them up to date. The indications for myocardial perfusion and coronary flow reserve contrast studies are discussed. Illustrative cases are included from a selection of centres experienced with the techniques as well as from the authors' own practice. Considerable attention is given to interpretation of the images and commonly encountered artifacts.

The final chapter introduces the more advanced topics of quantitative analysis of contrast images, including the estimation of relative myocardial vascular volume, flow velocity and perfusion rate. Examples are provided using software tools currently available for clinical use. An extensive index and a glossary of some of the many new terms used in contrast echocardiography are provided.

We believe that contrast agents have the potential to add an entirely new dimension to the role of ultrasound imaging in cardiology. If this book helps stimulate the reader to consider their use, it will have served its purpose.

Harald Becher
Peter N Burns

Bonn and Toronto, May 2000

Table of Contents

Foreword V

Preface VII

Table of Contents VII

Acknowledgements XIV

Chapter 1
Contrast agents for echocardiography: Principles and Instrumentation

1.1   The need for contrast agents in echocardiography 2
    1.1.1   B-mode imaging 2
    1.1.2   Doppler 3
    1.1.3   Doppler examination of small vessels 4

1.2   Contrast agents for ultrasound 5
    1.2.1   Contrast agent types 5
        1.2.1.1   Blood pool agents
        1.2.1.2   Selective uptake agents
    1.2.2   Using a contrast agent 8
        1.2.2.1   Preparation
        1.2.2.2   Preparing for injection
    1.2.3   Administration methods 12
        1.2.3.1   Bolus
        1.2.3.2   Infusion

1.3   Mode of action 16
    1.3.1   Bubble behaviour and incident pressure 17

   1.3.1.1 The Mechanical Index (MI)
  1.3.2 I – Linear Backscatter: Doppler enhancement 18
   1.3.2.1 Enhancement studies with conventional imaging
  1.3.3 II – Nonlinear backscatter: harmonic imaging 20
   1.3.3.1 The need for bubble-specific imaging
   1.3.3.2 Harmonic imaging
   1.3.3.3 The impact of harmonic imaging
   1.3.3.4 Tissue harmonic imaging
   1.3.3.5 Pulse inversion imaging
   1.3.3.6 Power pulse inversion imaging
  1.3.4 III – Transient disruption: intermittent imaging 36
   1.3.4.1 Triggered imaging
   1.3.4.2 Intermittent harmonic power Doppler
  1.3.5 Summary 39

1.4 Safety considerations 40

1.5 New developments in contrast imaging 41
  1.5.1 Tissue specific bubbles 41
  1.5.2 Bubbles for therapy 41

1.6 Summary 42

1.7 References 42

Chapter 2
Assessment of Left Ventricular Function by Contrast Echo

2.1 Physiology and pathophysiology of LV function 48

2.2 Available methods – The role of contrast 49
  2.2.1 Systolic function: the need for endocardial border definition 49
  2.2.2 Diastolic function: the need for pulmonary venous flow recordings 50

2.3 Indications and selection of methods 51
  2.3.1 Indications for contrast echo 51
   2.3.1.1 LV border delineation
   2.3.1.2 Detection, determination of size and shape of LV thrombi
   2.3.1.3 Pulmonary venous flow
  2.3.2 Selection of patients 53
  2.3.3 Selection of imaging methods 54

2.4 How to perform an LV contrast study 56
2.4.1 Fundamental B-mode 56
2.4.1.1 Contrast agent dose
2.4.1.2 Image acquisition and interpretation
2.4.1.3 Pitfalls and troubleshooting
2.4.2 Fundamental pulsed wave (PW)Doppler 59
2.4.2.1 Contrast agent dose
2.4.2.2 Image acquisition and interpretation
2.4.2.3 Pitfalls and troubleshooting
2.4.3 Harmonic B-mode 63
2.4.3.1 Contrast agent dose
2.4.3.2 Image acquisition and interpretation
2.4.3.3 Pitfalls and troubleshooting
2.4.4 Harmonic imaging of LV thrombi 67
2.4.5 Harmonic colour/power Doppler for LVO 68
2.4.5.1 Continuous imaging for evaluation of LV wall motion
2.4.5.2 Contrast agent dose
2.4.5.3 Image acquisition and interpretation
2.4.5.4 Pitfalls and troubleshooting
2.4.6 Triggered imaging for assessment of end-systolic and end-diastolic volumes and ejection fraction 72
2.4.6.1 Contrast agent dose
2.4.6.2 Image acquisition and interpretation
2.4.6.3 Pitfalls and troubleshooting

2.5 Summary 77

2.6 References 78

Chapter 3
Assessment of Myocardial Perfusion by Contrast Echo

3.1 Physiology and pathophysiology of myocardial perfusion 82
3.1.1 Normal perfusion 82
3.1.2 Acute myocardial infarction 83
3.1.3 Chronic ischemic heart disease 83

3.2 Currently available methods for myocardial perfusion imaging 84
3.2.1 Stress ECG 84
3.2.2 Stress echo 84

3.2.3	Coronary flow reserve (CFR)		85
3.2.4	Myocardial scintigraphy		85
3.2.5	Myocardial contrast echo		86

3.3 Indications and selection of methods ... 86
- 3.3.1 Indications ... 86
- 3.3.2 Selection of patients and contraindications ... 88
- 3.3.3 Selection of the imaging method ... 88
  - 3.3.3.1 Harmonic power Doppler (HPD)
  - 3.3.3.2 Harmonic B-Mode
  - 3.3.3.3 Pulse inversion imaging
  - 3.3.3.4 Power pulse inversion (PPI)

3.4 Special considerations for myocardial contrast ... 92
- 3.4.1 Impact of the scanplane ... 92
- 3.4.2 Triggered imaging ... 94
  - 3.4.2.1 Incremental triggered imaging
  - 3.4.2.2 Double or multiple trigger
  - 3.4.2.3 Flash echo
  - 3.4.2.4 Power pulse inversion flash echo
  - 3.4.2.5 Systolic versus diastolic trigger

3.5 Choice of agent and method of administration ... 97
- 3.5.1 Continuous infusion versus bolus injection ... 97
- 3.5.2 Preparation of contrast infusion ... 99
- 3.5.3 Adjustment of infusion rate ... 99

3.6 Instrument settings ... 100
- 3.6.1 Harmonic power Doppler ... 100
  - 3.6.1.1 Setting the trigger point
- 3.6.2 Harmonic B-mode ... 103
- 3.6.3 Pulse inversion imaging ... 106
- 3.6.4 Power pulse inversion ... 108

3.7 Image acquisition ... 108

3.8 Stress testing during myocardial contrast echo ... 109
- 3.8.1 Exercise and dobutamine stress ... 109
- 3.8.2 Vasodilator stress ... 109
- 3.8.3 Combined assessment of wall motion and myocardial perfusion ... 111

3.9 Reading myocardial contrast echocardiograms ... 112

3.9.1 Visual assessment of unprocessed recordings 112
    3.9.1.1 Normal perfusion
    3.9.1.2 Perfusion Defect
3.9.2 Visual assessment of post-processed recordings 119
3.9.3 Report of visual judgement 119

3.10 Clinical profiles/interpretation of myocardial contrast echo 121
3.10.1 Acute myocardial infarction 121
3.10.2 Scar or fibrosis versus viable myocardium 123
3.10.3 Coronary artery stenosis 124

3.11 Pitfalls and troubleshooting 127
3.11.1 Inadequate myocardial contrast 127
3.11.2 Contrast shadowing 129
3.11.3 Blooming 131
3.11.4 Wall motion artifacts 131
3.11.5 The bubble depletion artifact 133

3.12 Coronary flow reserve and myocardial contrast echo 133
3.12.1 What is coronary flow reserve? 134

3.13 Available methods – need for contrast enhancement 134

3.14 Coronary flow reserve: indications and selection of methods 135
3.14.1 Selection of patients 136

3.15 How to perform a CFR study 137
3.15.1 Intravenous lines 137
3.15.2 Contrast agent 137
3.15.3 Protocols to induce hyperemia 137
3.15.4 Image orientation for visualising blood flow in the LAD 139
3.15.5 Instrument settings 139
3.15.6 Combination with myocardial contrast echo (MCE) 141

3.16 Image acquisition and interpretation 142
3.16.1 Significance of an LAD stenosis 143
3.16.2 Follow-up of an LAD stenosis after PTCA 143

3.17 Pitfalls and troubleshooting 143
3.17.1 Angle of the vessel to the beam 143
3.17.2 Displacement of the sample volume 144
3.17.3 Flow in mammary artery 144

3.17.4	Bubble noise	145
3.17.5	Interpretation problems: impact of preload	146
3.17.6	Impact of blood pressure	146
3.17.7	Vasodilation during hyperemia	147

3.18 Summary 147

3.19 References 147

Chapter 4
Methods for quantitative Analysis

4.1 Basic tools for image quantification 154
    4.1.1 Single image quantification 155
    4.1.2 Cineloop quantification 156
        4.1.2.1 Reduction of data
        4.1.2.2 Positioning Regions of Interest (ROI)
        4.1.2.3 Automatic analysis

4.2 Advanced image processing: cases & examples 159
    4.2.1 Single image quantification 159
    4.2.2 Background subtraction 160
    4.2.3 Analysing the time-course of enhancement 164
        4.2.3.1 Intravenous bolus technique
        4.2.3.2 Negative bolus technique
        4.2.3.3 Real-time negative bolus technique

4.3 Summary 170

4.4 References 170

Glossary 172

Index 180

Acknowledgements

This book arose out of a series of seminars on contrast echocardiography organised by Sabino Iliceto of the University of Cagliari. We are grateful to Sabino and his colleagues, especially Carlo Caiati, for this and their contribution to the section on coronary flow reserve. We are also indebted to Danny Skyba and to Damien Dolimier, both pioneers of quantitative analysis of contrast echocardiograms, for their material which comprises much of Chapter 4. At home, we both acknowledge the invaluable help of our own colleagues: in Bonn, of Melanie Hümmelgen, Stefanie Kuntz, Heyder Omran, Birgit Piel, Rami Rabahieh, Rainer Schimpf, Klaus Tiemann; and in Toronto, of Cash Chin, Stuart Foster, Kasia Harasewicz, David Hope Simpson, Jennifer Lee Wah, Zvi Margaliot, Carrie Purcell, Howard and Sylvie.

Considerable effort was expended to produce a book which is easy to read and whose technical quality does justice to that of its many clinical images. The evident success is entirely that of Raffaela Kluge of Schering AG and Kay Bengelsdorf of Agentur B&S, who carried the production editing, typesetting and printing in Berlin, virtually single-handed. Their extraordinary efforts went far beyond these traditional roles and were supported by Luis Reimer Hevia of Schering and Walter Schimmel of B&S, to whom we are also grateful.

Finally, credibility is lent to a new clinical technique only when it is mastered by a large number of independent investigators; the authors are fortunate that the field of echocardiography is occupied by clinicians who are not only skilled and experienced, but open to innovation and dedicated to teaching. In this spirit a large number of them have contributed their own cases as illustrations to the contrast techniques described here. This handbook could not have been written without them, and we thank them all for their generosity:

Luciano Agati
University of Rome, Italy

Gian Paolo Bezante
University of Genoa, Italy

Carlo Caiati
University of Cagliari, Italy

Damien Dolimier
ATL Ultrasound, Bothell WA, USA

Steve Feinstein
Rush University, Chicago, USA

Kathy Ferrara
University of California, Davis, USA

Acknowledgment

Christian Firschke
University of Munich, Germany

Francesco Gentile
University of Milan, Italy

Sabino Iliceto
University of Cagliari, Italy

Sanjiv Kaul
University of Virginia, USA

Heinz Lambertz
Deutsche Klinik für Diagnostik, Wiesbaden, Germany

Roberto Lang
University of Chicago, USA

Jonathan Lindner
University of Virginia, USA

Thomas Marwick
University of Brisbane, Australia

Gerd P Meyer
University of Hanover, Germany

Mark Monaghan
University of London, UK

Sharon Mulvagh
Mayo Clinic, USA

Thomas Porter
University of Nebraska, USA

Ricardo Ronderos
Universidad Nacional de La Plata, Argentina

Jiri Sklenar
University of Virginia, USA

Danny Skyba
ATL Ultrasound, Bothell WA, USA

Folkert Ten Cate
Thorax Centre, Rotterdam, Netherlands

Jim Thomas
Cleveland Clinic, USA

Neil Weissman
Washington Hospital, Washington DC, USA

Eric Yu
University of Toronto, Canada

J Luis Zamorano
University of Madrid, Spain

1 Contrast Agents for Echocardiography: Principles and Instrumentation

Shall I refuse my dinner because I do not fully understand the process of digestion?

Oliver Heaviside, 1850–1925

Introduction

Contrast agents for ultrasound are unique in that they interact with, and form part of, the imaging process. Contrast imaging cannot be performed effectively without a basic understanding of this interaction and how it is exploited by the new imaging modes that have become available on modern ultrasound systems. In this chapter we consider how echocardiography might benefit from a contrast agent, describe currently available agents and explain their mode of action. We discuss the impact of ultrasound contrast on echocardiographic techniques and instrumentation and conclude with the most recent developments in this rapidly evolving field.

1.1 The need for contrast agents in echocardiography

1.1.1 B-mode imaging

It is well known that blood appears 'black' on ultrasound imaging. This is not because blood produces no echo, it is simply that the sound scattered by red blood cells at the low diagnostic frequencies is very weak, about 1,000–10,000 times weaker than that from solid tissue, so lies below the displayed dynamic range of the image. Amongst the roles that the image plays in the ultrasound examination of the heart is the identification of boundaries, especially of those between the blood and the wall of the cavity. Identification of the entire margin of the endocardium in a view of the left ventricle, for example, is an important component of any wall motion study. Although in some patients this boundary is seen clearly, in many the endocardial border is poorly defined because of the presence of spurious echoes within the cavity. These echoes, which are frequently a result of reverberation of the ultrasound beam between the transducer and the chest wall and aberration of the beam in its path between the ribs, result in a reduction of useful contrast between the wall and the cavity – the blurred haze that is familiar to many ultrasonographers. By enhancing the echo from blood in these patients by using a contrast agent, the blood in the cavity can be rendered visible above these artifacts. Because it is more homogeneous than the wall and because it is flowing, this echo does not suffer from the same artifacts and a clear boundary is seen, revealing the border of the endocardium (Figure 1).

If the echo from blood is enhanced by a contrast agent, the signals obtained from a duplex Doppler examination of the vessel will be similarly enhanced (Figure 2). A further role for such an agent immediately suggests itself. If the echo from large blood vessels can be

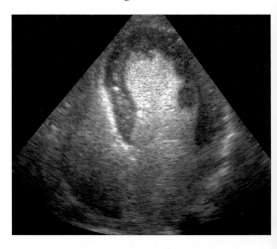

Fig. 1 Contrast enhanced harmonic image of the left ventricle shows the endocardial border clearly.

Principles and Instrumentation

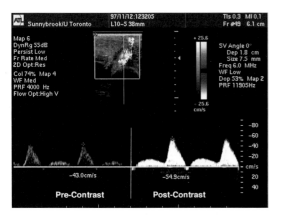

Fig. 2 Enhancement of Doppler signals by a microbubble contrast agent. The spectral display shows an increase in intensity with the arrival of the agent in an artery following intravenous injection.

enhanced by an agent, what effect will it have on the small volume of blood that is in the microvessels of the myocardium? The muscle itself appears bright on an ultrasound image, so we can expect the additional brightness due to the agent in the myocardial vessels to be very small, yet if it is detectable, it would open the possibility of using ultrasound to map the relative perfusion volume of blood in the muscle itself. As we shall see, it is normally not possible to detect this tiny echo with existing techniques, but with the aid of new methods such as harmonic and pulse inversion imaging and Doppler, myocardial perfusion volume imaging becomes possible with ultrasound.

Contrast in echocardiography: why?

- To enhance Doppler flow signals from the cavities and great vessels
- To delineate the endocardium by cavity opacification
- To image perfusion in the myocardium

1.1.2 Doppler

Doppler forms an essential part of all echocardiography examinations. It is used both to detect large volumes of blood moving slowly, such as in the cavities, and small volumes of blood moving fast, such as in stenotic valvular jets. It is also used in many vascular beds to visualise the flow at the parenchymal level of the circulation, where blood vessels lie below the resolvable limit of the image. The detection of such 'unresolved' flow using Doppler systems can be demonstrated simply by using a duplex scanner to create a power Doppler image of an abdominal organ such as the kidney, in which vessels that are not seen on the greyscale image become visible using the Doppler mode. These vessels are the arcuate and interlobular branches of the renal artery, whose diameter is known to be less than 100 μm and therefore below the resolution limit of the image. However, as we progress distally in the arterial system, the blood flows more slowly as the rate of bifurcation increases, producing lower Doppler shift frequencies. The quantity of blood in a given volume of tissue also decreases, weakening the backscattered echo. Eventually, a point is reached at which the vessel cannot be visualised and the Doppler signals cannot be detected. The myocardial perfusion bed lies beyond this point.

Conditions for successful Doppler detection of blood flow

- Velocity of flow must be sufficient to give detectable Doppler shift
- Strength of blood echo must be sufficient for detection
- Tissue motion must be sufficiently slow that its Doppler shift may be distinguished from that of blood flow

1.1.3 Doppler examination of small vessels

To understand how contrast agents may help to image myocardial perfusion we need to examine these performance limits for the Doppler detection of blood flow. Two conditions must be satisfied before a Doppler signal can be detected: first, the velocity of blood must be sufficient to produce a Doppler shift frequency that is distinguishable from that produced by the normal motion of tissue, and second, the strength of the echo must provide a sufficient signal at the transducer to allow detection above the acoustic and electrical noise of the system. For fast moving blood, such as that in a stenotic jet, it is the second condition that determines if a Doppler interrogation – in spectral or colour modes – fails to obtain a signal. If the echo is too weak, the examination fails. The role of the contrast agent is to enhance the blood echo, thereby increasing the signal-to-noise ratio and hence the success rate of a Doppler examination. Figure 3 shows how with the addition of a contrast agent, a colour Doppler system can show the apical coronary vessels from a transthoracic view.

For small blood vessels, on the other hand, the diagnostic objective in using an ultrasound contrast agent is to detect flow in the circulation at a level that is lower than would otherwise be possible in Doppler or greyscale modes. In cardiac applications the target small vessels are those supplying the myocardium. The echoes from blood associated with such flow – at the arteriolar level for example – exist in the midst of echoes from the surrounding solid structures of the organ parenchyma, echoes which are almost always stronger than even the contrast-enhanced blood echo. Thus, in order

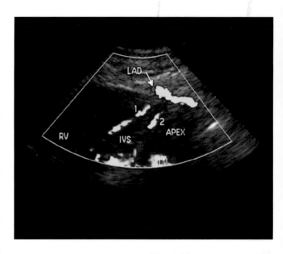

Fig. 3 Contrast enhanced Doppler examiniation of the apical coronary vessels.

to be able to image flow in the myocardium, a contrast agent is required that either increases the blood echo to a level that is substantially higher than that of the surrounding tissue, or a method must be conceived for suppressing the echo from non-contrast-bearing structures. Although Doppler is an effective method for separating the echoes from blood and tissue, it relies on the relatively high velocity of the flowing blood compared to that of, say, the cardiac wall. Although this distinction – which allows us to use a highpass (or 'wall') filter to separate the Doppler signals due to bloodflow from those due to the wall itself – is valid for flow in large vessels or across the cardiac valves, it is not valid for the myocardium, where the muscle is moving much faster than the blood which flows in its vasculature. Thus the Doppler shift frequency from the moving muscle is comparable to or higher than that of the moving blood itself. Because the wall filter cannot be used without eliminating both the flow and the muscle echoes, the use of Doppler in such circumstances is defeated by the overwhelming signal from tissue movement: the

Principles and Instrumentation

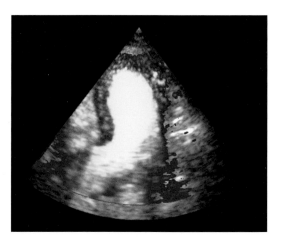

Fig. 4 Myocardial perfusion imaged using intermittent harmonic power Doppler and Levovist.

'flash' artifact in colour or the 'thump' artifact in spectral Doppler. Thus myocardial flow cannot be imaged with conventional Doppler, with or without intravenous contrast agents. A new Doppler modality is necessary: as we shall see, harmonic and pulse inversion imaging provide this (Figure 4).

1.2 Contrast agents for ultrasound

The principal requirements for an ultrasound contrast agent are that it should be easily introducible into the vascular system, be stable for the duration of the diagnostic examination, have low toxicity and modify one or more acoustic properties of tissues which determine the ultrasound imaging process. Although it is conceivable that applications may be found for ultrasound contrast agents which will justify their injection directly into arteries, the clinical context for contrast ultrasonography requires that they be capable of intravenous administration. As we shall see, these constitute a demanding specification for a drug, one that only recently has been met. The technology universally adopted is that of encapsulated bubbles of gas which are smaller than red blood cells and therefore capable of circulating freely in the body. These are the so-called 'blood pool' agents. Agents have also been conceived that are taken up by a chosen organ system or site, as are many nuclear medicine materials.

An ideal ultrasound contrast agent

- Non-toxic
- Intravenously injectable, by bolus or infusion
- Stable during cardiac and pulmonary passage
- Remains within the blood pool or has a well-specified tissue distribution
- Duration of effect comparable to that of the imaging examination

1.2.1 Contrast agent types

Contrast agents might act by their presence in the vascular system, from where they are ultimately metabolised ('blood pool' agents) or by their selective uptake in tissue after a vascular phase. Of the properties of tissue that influence the ultrasound image, the most important are backscatter coefficient, attenuation and acoustic propagation velocity (1). Most agents seek to enhance the echo by increasing the backscatter of the tissue that bears them as much as possible, while increasing the attenuation in the tissue as little as possible, thus enhancing the echo from blood.

1.2.1.1 Blood pool agents

Free gas bubbles

Gramiak and Shah first used injected bubbles to enhance the blood pool echo in 1968 (2). They injected saline into the ascending aorta during echocardiographic recording and noted strong echoes within the normally echo free lumen of the aorta and the chambers of the heart. Subsequent work showed that these reflections were the result of free bubbles of air which came out of solution either by agitation or by cavitation during the injection itself. In this early work, many other fluids were found to produce a contrast effect when similarly injected (3, 4). The intensity of the echoes produced varied with the type of solution used: the more viscous the solution, the more microbubbles were trapped in a bolus for a sufficient length of time to be appreciated on the image. Agitated solutions of compounds such as indocyanine green and renografin were also used.

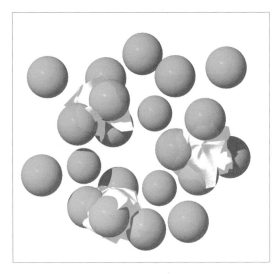

Fig. 5 The principle of Levovist. Air adheres to the surface of galactose microparticles which 'size' the resulting bubbles to have a median diameter of about 4 µm. Upon dissolution, the bubbles are coated with a thin, permeable shell comprising palmitic acid.

Most of the subsequent research into the application of these bubbles as ultrasound contrast agents focused on the heart, including evaluation of valvular insufficiency (5, 6), intracardiac shunts (7) and cavity dimensions (8). The fundamental limitation of bubbles produced in this way is that they are large, so that they are effectively filtered by the lungs, and unstable, so that they go back into solution within a second or so. Hence this procedure was invasive and, except by direct injection, unsuitable for imaging of left-sided cardiac chambers, the coronary circulation and the systemic arterial tree and its organs.

Encapsulated air bubbles

To overcome the natural instability of free gas bubbles, attempts were made to encapsulate gas within a shell so as to create a more stable particle. In 1980 Carroll et al (9) encapsulated nitrogen bubbles in gelatin and injected them into the femoral artery of rabbits with VX2 tumours in the thigh. Ultrasound enhancement of the tumour rim was identified. However, the large size of the particles (80 µm) precluded administration by an intravenous route. The challenge to produce a stable encapsulated microbubble of a comparable size to that of a red blood cell and which could survive passage through the heart and the pulmonary capillary network was first met by Feinstein et al in 1984 (10), who produced microbubbles by sonication of a solution of human serum albumin and showed that it could be visualised in the left heart after a peripheral venous injection. This agent was subsequently developed commercially as Albunex® (Mallinckrodt Medical Inc, St Louis, MO).

A burgeoning number of manufacturers have since produced forms of stabilised microbubbles that are currently being assessed for use as intravenous contrast agents for ultrasound. Several have passed through 'Phase 3' clinical trials and gained regulatory approval in Europe, North America and, more recently, Japan. Levovist® (Schering AG, Berlin, Germany), is a dry mixture comprising 99.9 percent microcrystalline galactose microparticles, and 0.1 percent palmitic acid. Upon dissolution and agitation in sterile water, the galactose disaggregates into microparticles which provide an irregular surface for the adherence of microbubbles 3 to 4 μm in size (Figure 5). Stabilisation of the microbubbles takes place as they become coated with palmitic acid, which separates the gas – liquid interface and slows their dissolution (11). These microbubbles are highly echogenic and are sufficiently stable for transit through the pulmonary circuit. The estimated median particle size is 1.8 μm and the median bubble diameter approximately 2 μm with the 97th centile approximately 6 μm (12). The agent is chemically related to its predecessor Echovist® (Schering AG, Berlin, Germany) a galactose agent that forms larger bubbles and which has been used extensively without suggestion of toxicity. Both preclinical (13) and clinical (14) studies with Levovist demonstrate its capacity to traverse the pulmonary bed in sufficient concentrations to enhance both colour Doppler and, in some instances, the B-mode image itself.

Low solubility gas bubbles
The 'shells' which stabilise the microbubbles are extremely thin and allow a gas such as air to diffuse out and go back into solution in the blood. How fast this happens depends on a number of factors which have been seen to vary not only from agent to agent, but from patient to patient. After venous introduction, however, the effective duration of the two agents described above is of the order of a few minutes. Because they are introduced as a bolus and the maximum effect of the agent is in the first pass, the useful imaging time is usually considerably less than this. Newer (sometimes referred to as 'second generation') agents, designed both to increase backscatter enhancement further and to last longer in the bloodstream are currently under development and early clinical use. Instead of air, many of these take advantage of low solubility gases such as perfluorocarbons, the consequent lower diffusion rate increasing the longevity of the agent in the blood. However, a price may be paid for this stability in the reduced acoustic responsiveness of the agent (see §1.3.4.2). Optison® (Mallinckrodt Medical Inc, St Louis, MO) is a perfluoropropane filled albumin shell with a size distribution similar to that of Albunex (Figure 6). The stability of the smaller bubbles in its population is the probable cause of the greater enhancement observed with this agent. Echogen® (Sonus Inc, Bothell WA) is an emulsion of dodecafluoropentane droplets which undergo a phase change, 'boiling' to create gas which is stabilised into bubbles by an accompanying surfactant. In practice, this

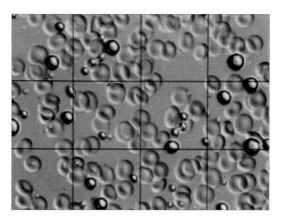

Fig. 6 Optison microbubbles photographed in vitro with red blood cells (Courtesy Mallinckrodt Inc).

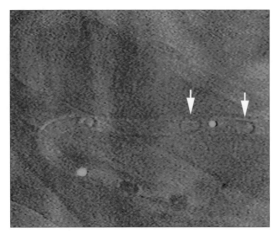

Fig. 7 Definity microbubbles seen flowing in a blood vessel. Intravital microscopy shows a capillary following intravenous administration of fluorescent-labeled agent. Two microbubbles traverse the vessel with adjacent red blood cells (arrows) seen faintly under the concomitant low-level trans-illumination.
Courtesy Jonathan Lindner, University of Virginia, VA, USA

agent requires external preparation of the mixture (eg, the 'popping' of a syringe by forced withdrawing of the plunger against its closed outlet) to create the bubble population before injection. SonoVue™ (Bracco Inc, NJ) uses sulphur hexafluorane in a phosphorlipid shell. Definity™ (also known as DMP115, DuPont Inc, Boston MA) comprises a perfluoropropane microbubble coated with a particularly flexible bilipid shell which also shows improved stability and high enhancements at low doses (15) (Figure 7). Other agents are under aggressive development (see Table).

1.2.1.2 Selective uptake agents

A perfect blood pool agent displays the same flow dynamics as blood itself, and is ultimately metabolised from the blood pool. Agents can be made, however, that are capable of providing ultrasound contrast during their metabolism as well as while in the blood pool. Colloidal suspensions of liquids such as perfluorocarbons (16) and certain agents with durable shells (17) are taken up by the reticuloendothelial system from where they ultimately are excreted. There they may provide contrast from within the liver parenchyma, demarking the distribution of Kupffer cells (18). In the future, such agents with a cell-specific pathway may be used as a means both to detect and to deliver therapeutic agents to a specific site in the cardiovascular system.

1.2.2 Using a contrast agent

There is no question that the majority of difficulties that occur when a contrast agent is first used in a clinical echo laboratory can be attributed to problems with the preparation and administration of the injected material itself. Many physicians and nurses used to administering pharmaceutical drugs, including x-ray contrast, cannot understand why the preparation and injection itself are so critical for

The evolution of contrast agents for ultrasound		
'Generation'	Formulation	Characteristics
0	Free gas bubbles	Could not traverse cardiopulmonary beds
1	Encapsulated air bubbles	Successful trans-pulmonary passage
2	Encapsulated low solubility gas bubbles	Improved stability
3	'Particulate' (eg polymer shell) gas bubbles	Controlled acoustic properties

Some ultrasound contrast agents

Manufacturer	Name	Type	Development Stage
Acusphere	AI-700	Polymer/perflourocarbon	Early Development
Alliance/Schering	Imavist™	Surfactant/perfluorohexane-air	Clinical Development
Bracco	SonoVue™	Phospholipid/Sulphur hexafluoride	Late Clinical Development
Byk-Gulden	BY963	Lipid/air	Not commercially developed
Cavcon	Filmix™	Lipid/air	Pre-clinical Development
DuPont	Definity™	Liposome/perfluoropropane	Late Clinical Development
Molecular Biosystems/Mallinckrodt	Optison®	Cross-linked human serum albumin/perfluoropropane	Approved in EU, US, Canada
Molecular Biosystems/Mallinckrodt	Albunex®	Sonicated albumin/air	Approved in EU, US
Nycomed	Sonazoid™	Lipid/perfluorocarbon	Late Clinical Development
Point Biomedical	Bisphere™	Polymer bilayer/air	Clinical Development
Porter	PESDA	Sonicated dextrose albumin/perfluorocarbon	Not commercially developed
Quadrant	Quantison™	Spray-dried albumin/air	Pre-clinical Development
Schering	Echovist®	Galactose matrix/air	Approved in EU, Canada
Schering	Levovist®	Lipid/air	Approved in 69 countries, including EU, Canada, Japan (not US)
Schering	Sonavist™	Polymer/air	Clinical Development
Sonus Pharmaceutical	Echogen®	Surfactant/dodecafluoropentane	Late Clinical Development

an ultrasound contrast study. Yet although they are classified as drugs, all current agents are really physical suspensions of bubbles in an inactive medium such as saline. The bubbles are stabilised by shells that are sometimes only tens of nanometres in thickness: they are physically delicate and particularly susceptible to destruction by pressure or shear stress. The gas also diffuses out of the bubbles with time and sometimes this process is faster outside the body than once injected. In addition, the bubbles have a tendency to float and hence separate from the solution that holds them over a period of time. As long as it is realised the bubble suspensions cannot be handled like an ordinary drug and require special care, it is relatively easy to prepare the echo laboratory for their handling.

1.2.2.1 Preparation

It should be appreciated that no two agents are alike in the way that they are prepared for injection. Some vials contain bubbles that simply are reconstituted by the addition of saline, others rely on the user to manufacture the bubbles during the preparation process. These require mechanical agitation or a more elaborate mixing procedure that must be followed carefully.

Levovist is prepared by injection of sterile water into a vial containing a sugar/lipid powder followed by vigorous shaking of the vial by hand. The agent can be administered in one of three concentrations (200, 300 or 400 mg/ml), upon which the volume of water to be used depends. It should be left to stand for about 2 minutes after mixing. The more concentrated suspensions are somewhat viscous, so that bubble flotation is not a practical problem with this agent. The bubbles are, however, sensitive to the increase of pressure within the vial that would result from the injection of the water into a closed space, so the vial is vented for the addition of water and withdrawal of the agent by the use of a special cap provided with each dose (Figure 8). The agent should be used within about 30 minutes of preparation.

Optison is kept in a refrigerator from which it should be removed to bring it to room temperature before use. It is prepared by simple shaking by hand and withdrawal from a vented vial through an 18-gauge needle. Optison bubbles are buoyant and have a tendency to rise quickly to the surface of the syringe unless it is gently but constantly rotated before injection.

SonoVue is prepared by simple mixing with saline, which is provided in the measured syringe kit (Figure 9). The bubbles are also

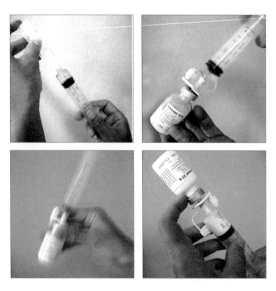

Fig. 8 Preparation of Levovist. Sterile water is measured according to the concentration required and added to a vial of dry powder through a special venting cap. The mixture is agitated by hand and left to stand for two minutes before slow withdrawal into the injecting syringe through the cap.

Principles and Instrumentation

buoyant and the preparation of quite low viscosity, so the bubbles also float rapidly. SonoVue can be infused effectively using an infusion pump, but care should be taken to ensure that the direction of the infused output is vertical, so that bubbles do not become trapped.

Definity, like Optison, is already mixed when the vial is manufactured. However, the bubbles are formed only after the vial has been agitated for 45 seconds in a mechanical shaker, which is most conveniently located in the examination room (Figure 10 a, b). The agent is withdrawn from the vial by venting with a second 18-gauge needle and may be injected by syringe (Figure 10 c) or infused by simple injection into a drip bag (Figure 10 d). In this form Definity is unusually stable and the bubbles neutrally buoyant, so that flotation is not a problem.

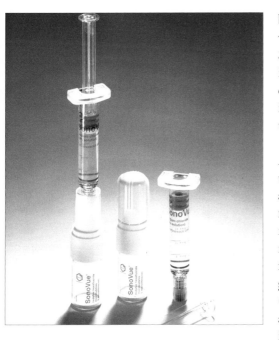

Fig. 9 Preparation of SonoVue. The agent is packaged as a dry powder and reconstituted using saline measured in a the syringe supplied.

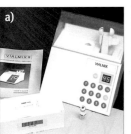
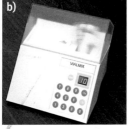
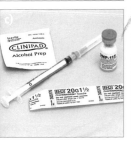
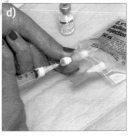

Fig. 10 Preparation of Definity. The vial is agitated by a mechanical device supplied specifically for this agent (a, b). It is then withdrawn from the vial for bolus injection (c) or injected directly into a drip bag for infusion (d).

Preparing a contrast agent: tips

- Establish machine settings and scan patient before mixing the agent
- Use vents: never withdraw from or inject agent against a closed space
- Watch for flotation of bubbles: gently shake the vial and syringe after preparation
- Follow the manufacturer's directions carefully

1.2.2.2 Preparing for injection

With all agents, the use of smaller diameter needles should be avoided because the bubbles are subjected to large pressure drop due to the Bernoulli effect as the fluid exits the tip of the lumen. The faster the injection and the smaller the diameter, the larger the pressure drop and the greater the likelihood of damage to the bubbles. A 22-gauge or larger needle is best. It should be borne in mind that the smaller the

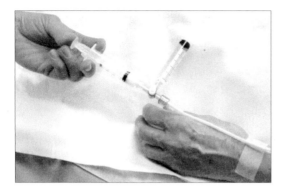

Fig. 11 A three way stopcock, line and flush ready for injection of Optison.

needle lumen, the slower the injection should be to avoid inadvertent bubble destruction. Bubbles can also be destroyed by pushing the syringe plunger against a closed line: if this happens accidentally, the dose should be discarded. Because the total injection volume for some studies can be less than 1ml, a flush is needed to push the agent into the central venous stream. 5–10 ml saline administered through a 3-way stopcock at the end of a short line which allows free movement of the syringe for mixing is often best. It is good practice for the saline to traverse the right angle bend of the stopcock, not the agent, which should be connected along the direct path, again to avoid bubble destruction (Figure 11).

Administering a contrast agent: tips

- Establish the venous line before preparing the agent
- Use a 22-gauge or larger cannulation; cubital vein is often best
- Use a 3-way stopcock if preferred but never push filled syringe against a closed valve
- Watch for bubble flotation: keep the syringe moving between injections
- Inject slowly: follow the manufacturer's recommendations

1.2.3 Administration methods

1.2.3.1 Bolus

Figure 12 shows dose-response measurements made using a dedicated Doppler probe positioned on the brachial artery of a patient after an injection of Optison. A first-pass peak enhancement of 30 dB is followed by a steady, exponential wash-out of about 3 minutes' duration, which is typical of the kinetics of a blood pool microbubble agent. The huge enhancement at the peak usually causes over-

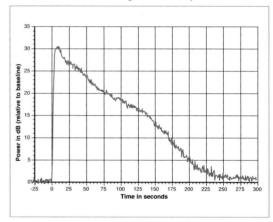

Fig. 12 Example of typical time enhancement curve measured in the brachial artery of a patient after injection with Optison. Note that the effective duration of enhancement in this case is about 3 minutes.

loading of the Doppler receiver, creating spectral or colour blooming. Sonographers commonly evade this by waiting until the wash-out phase, in which a more suitable enhancement can be obtained for a longer period. It is clear, however, that this is an inefficient way to use the agent because the majority of bubbles do not contribute to the collection of diagnostic information. Decreasing the bolus volume does not necessarily help. If the dose of Optison is increased progressively from

Principles and Instrumentation

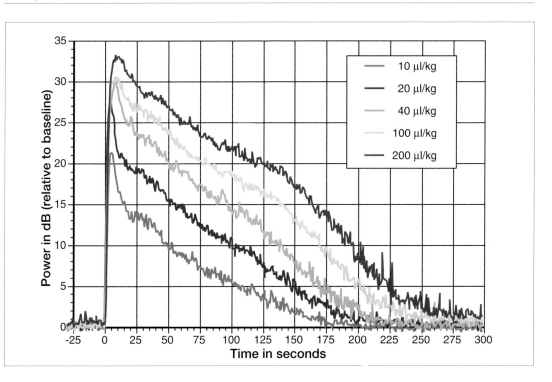

Fig. 13 The enhancement curves of Optison with increasing dose. Note that increasing the dose increases both the peak enhancement and the wash-out time of the agent.

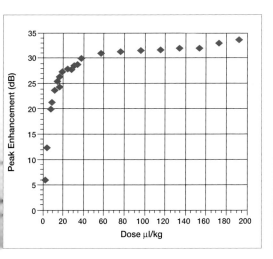

Fig. 14 Peak enhancement as a function of administered dose. This graph shows that the effect of the agent at its peak does not increase with large doses. This may be due to 'bolus spreading'.

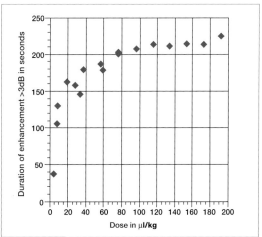

Fig. 15 Duration of enhancement as a function of administered dose. Note that the effect of larger doses is to extend the duration of enhancement, rather than increase the height of the peak effect.

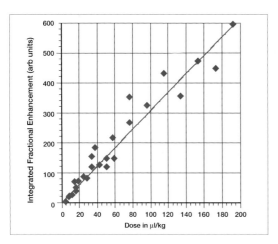

Fig. 16 Integrated fractional enhancement (defined as the area under the curves of Figure 13) plotted as a function of dose for Optison. A steadily increasing response is seen as the administered volume of the agent is increased.

10–200 µl/kg (Figure 13), we see the peak enhancement increase slightly and the wash-out time increase more dramatically. Note that increasing the dose by a factor of 10 does not have the same effect on the peak enhancement (Figure 14). Instead, it is the wash-out time of the agent, reflected by the duration of enhancement that is increased (Figure 15). The area under these curves represents the product of the enhancement and the time of enhancement and may be regarded as a crude measure of the integrated effect of the agent. If this is plotted against the dose we see (Figure 16) that increasing the volume of a bolus causes this value to rise in a roughly linear manner. It is on this observation that the effort to infuse agents is based.

1.2.3.2 Infusion

Although there is a definite role for bolus injection where short duration, maximum effect is required from the agent (eg in LV opacification for the wall motion studies of §2.4), infusing a contrast agent offers the possibility of enhancement for a length of time that more closely matches that of the imaging examination. Agents may be infused by slow injection, by use of an injection pump, by dripping the diluted agent through an IV line, or by use of an infusion pump of the kind used to titrate IV drugs. Figure 17 compares SonoVue administered as a bolus (Figure 17 a) and as an infusion through an IV pump (Figure 17 b). Figure 18 shows the results of a slow manual injection of Levovist, with an enhancement of 15 dB effectively lasting for more than 9 minutes. It can be seen that the effect of infusion is to maintain an enhancement comparable to that of the peak bolus for a period which matches more closely that of the clinical ultrasound examination. There is, then, a clear advantage to infusing contrast agents, not least of which is that the improved efficiency translates into an economic saving on the cost of the agent. Against this must be weighed a few practical considerations which vary from agent to agent.

First, if a slow or mechanically controlled injection is to be used, the agent must remain stable in the syringe for the duration of the infusion. Levovist, which is quite viscous after mixing,

Bolus: pros and cons	
Pro	Con
Easy to perform	Contrast effect short lived
Highest peak enhancement	Contrast effect changing during study
Wash-in and wash-out visible	Timing of bolus difficult
Agent is used quickly: no stability problems	Comparative contrast studies difficult

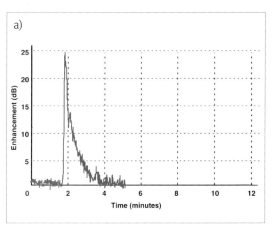
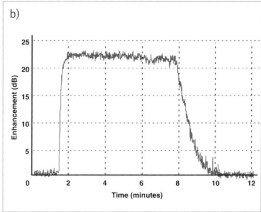

Fig. 17 Bolus vs infusion. (a) A bolus injection of SonoVue gives a wash-out time of about 1 minute. (b) Infused, the agent delivers uniform enhancement over a period of about 7 minutes.

provides this more easily than, say Optison, in which emulsion the bubbles tend to float. Agitating the preparation while it is in the syringe is in practice difficult. On the other hand, some perfluorocarbon agents such as Definity are effective in very high dilution, rendering them ideal for injection into a drip bag and drip infusion. This cannot be attempted with Levovist because of the adverse effect of dilution on the bubble population. Finally, some agents which are effective at very low volumes require whole body doses of much less

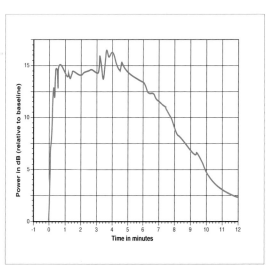

Fig. 18 The enhancement provided by a slow manual injection of Levovist. Enhancement is seen to last for approximately nine minutes.

Infusion: pros and cons	
Pro	Con
Extends time of enhancement	More complex to perform: may require pump
Provides consistent effect	Titration of infusion takes time and effort
Avoids blooming/ artifacts	Stability of agent over infusion period can be a problem
Dose is optimised: agent is used more efficiently	
Allows negative bolus method for quantitation of perfusion (see Ch4)	

than 1ml, rendering infusion difficult and slow injection virtually impossible. Others, which are fundamentally unstable out of the body, such as Echogen, offer no obvious means for infusion or slow injection. Clearly, the manufacturers' advice should be sought before attempting infusion in a clinical setting. The Table below shows when an infusion is sessential to contrast examination.

When is an infusion necessary?

Infusion mandatory	Bolus sufficient
Myocardial perfusion: rest and stress studies, quantitative analysis	Myocardial perfusion: rest studies only, qualitative assessment
Coronary flow reserve	LVO: rest or stress, thrombus detection
	Pulmonary vein Doppler enhancement

1.3 Mode of action

The interaction of an ultrasound beam with a population of bubbles is a process whose subtlety and complexity has only recently been recognised. Understanding what happens when a microbubble contrast agent is exposed to an ultrasound beam is the key to understanding – and using – new clinical methods for contrast imaging and thus the key to interpreting a clinical contrast echocardiographic study.

A sound field comprises a train of travelling waves, much like ripples on a pond. The fluid pressure of the medium (in this case tissue) changes as the sound propagates through it. A gas bubble is highly compliant and hence is squashed when the pressure outside it is raised and expanded when the pressure is lowered. At a typical clinical frequency of 2 MHz, for example, a bubble sitting in an acoustic field undergoes this oscillatory motion two million times per second. As it moves in this way, the bubble becomes a source of sound that radiates radially from its location in the body, as would

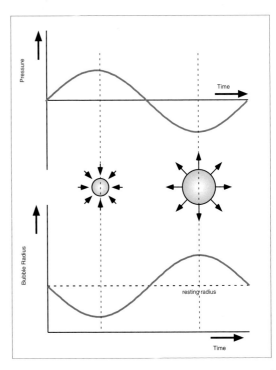

Fig. 19 A bubble in an acoustic field responds to the changes in pressure which constitute the sound wave by changing in size. The radius oscillates at the same rate as the incident sound, radiating an echo.

ripples on a pond from a small object moving at a point on its surface (Figure 19). The sound that reaches the transducer from this bubble, combined with that from all of its neighbours, is what constitutes the scattered echo from a contrast agent. Characterising this echo so that it can be differentiated from those of ordinary tissue such as the cardiac muscle is the basis of contrast specific imaging modes such as pulse inversion Doppler or harmonic imaging.

1.3.1 Bubble behaviour and incident pressure

Unlike tissue, a bubble does not scatter in the same way if it is exposed to weak (that is low amplitude) sound, than to strong, high amplitude sound. Instead, there are three broad regimes of scattering behaviour that depend on the peak pressure of the incident sound field produced by the scanner (see Table). These are used in different ways in contrast imaging of the heart.

Looking at the Table, we see that at low incident pressures (corresponding to low transmit power of the scanner), the agents produce linear backscatter enhancement, resulting in an augmentation of the echo from blood. This is the behaviour originally envisaged by the contrast agent manufacturers for their first intended clinical indication: Doppler signal enhancement. It is this for which they obtained approval from the regulatory authorities, an indication which does not require any change to ultrasound imaging and Doppler instrumentation. As the transmit intensity control of the scanner is increased and the pressure incident on a bubble goes beyond about 50–100 kPa, which is still below the level used in most diagnostic scans, the contrast agent backscatter begins to show nonlinear characteristics, such as the emission of harmonics. It is the detection of these that forms the basis of contrast specific imaging modes such as harmonic and pulse inversion imaging and Doppler. Finally, as the peak pressure passes about 1 MPa, near the maximum emitted by a typical echo imaging system, many agents exhibit transient nonlinear scattering. This forms the basis of triggered imaging and most strategies for detection of myocardial perfusion. The Table shows these three regimes together with the imaging methods developed to exploit them. It should be noted that in practice,

Three regimes of bubble behaviour in an ultrasound field

Peak pressure (approx)	Mechanical Index (MI) @ 1MHz	Bubble behaviour	Acoustic behaviour	Clinical Application
< 100 kPa	< 0.1	Linear oscillation	Backscatter enhancement	Coronary artery Doppler, PV Doppler, fundamental B-mode LVO
100 kPa–1 MPa	0.1 – 1.0	Nonlinear oscillation	Harmonic backscatter	Coronary artery Doppler, harmonic B-mode LVO, real-time perfusion imaging
> 1 MPa	> 1.0	Disruption	Transient harmonic echoes	Power Doppler LVO, intermittent perfusion imaging

because of the different sizes present in a realistic population of bubbles (19), the borders between these behaviours are not sharp. Nor will they be the same for different agent types, whose acoustic behaviour is strongly dependent on the gas and shell properties (20). In the next section we examine the clinical imaging methods which rely on each of these behaviours in turn.

1.3.1.1 The Mechanical Index (MI)

For reasons unrelated to contrast imaging, ultrasound scanners marketed in the US are required by the Food and Drugs Administration (FDA) to carry an on-screen label of the estimated peak negative pressure to which tissue is exposed. Of course, this pressure changes according to the tissue through which the sound travels as well as the amplitude and geometry of the ultrasound beam: the higher the attenuation, the less the peak pressure in tissue will be. A scanner cannot 'know' what tissue it is being used on, so the definition of an index has been arrived at which reflects the approximate exposure to ultrasound pressure at the focus of the beam in an average tissue. The Mechanical Index (or 'MI') is defined as the peak rarefactional (that is, negative) pressure, divided by the square root of the ultrasound frequency. This quantity is related to the amount of mechanical work that can be performed on a bubble during a single negative half cycle of sound (21). In clinical ultrasound systems, this index usually lies somewhere between 0.1 and 2.0. Although a single value is displayed for each image, in practice the actual MI varies throughout the image. In the absence of attenuation, the MI is maximal at the focus of the beam. Attenuation shifts this maximum towards the transducer. In a phased array, steering reduces the intensity of the ultrasound beam so that the MI is also less at the edges of the sector. Furthermore, because it is a somewhat complex procedure to calculate the index, which is itself only an estimate of the actual quantity within the body, the indices displayed by different machines are not precisely comparable. Thus, for example, more bubble disruption might be observed at a displayed MI of 1.0 using one machine than on the same patient using another. For this reason, recommendations of machine settings for a specific examination will include MI values peculiar to a given ultrasound manufacturer's instrument. Nonetheless, the MI is one of the most important machine parameters in a contrast echo study. It is usually controlled by means of the 'output power' setting of the scanner.

The Mechanical Index (MI)

- Defined by $MI = \frac{P_{neg}}{\sqrt{f}}$, where P_{neg} is the peak negative ultrasound pressure, f the ultrasound frequency
- Reflects the normalised energy to which a target (such as a bubble) is exposed in an ultrasound field
- Is defined for the focus of the ultrasound beam
- Varies with depth in the image (lessens with increasing depth)
- Varies with lateral location in the image (lessens towards the sector edges)

1.3.2 I – Linear backscatter: Doppler enhancement

Although bubbles of a typical contrast agent are smaller than red blood cells, and their volume concentration in the blood following intravenous injection is a fraction of a percent, the amplitude of the echo from the microbubble agent eclipses that of the blood itself.

This is because the weakness of the echo from blood originates from the cells themselves, which are poor scatterers of ultrasound. Their acoustic impedance is almost identical to that of the surrounding plasma. A bubble containing compressible gas, on the other hand, presents a strong discontinuity in acoustic impedance and hence acts as a strong reflector. Size for size, a bubble is about one hundred million million times more effective at scattering ultrasound. Thus the injection of a relatively sparse population of bubbles into the bloodstream results in a substantial enhancement of the blood echo. In a Doppler examination, the arrival of the contrast agent, some seconds after peripheral venous injection, in the portion of the systemic vasculature under interrogation is marked by a dramatic increase in signal strength. In spectral Doppler this is seen as an intensifying of the greyscale of the spectrum (Figure 2), whose enhancement is related to dose and whose duration depends on the method of administration. A 10 ml bolus of Levovist at a concentration of 400 mg/ml, for example, provides a peak enhancement of about 25 dB with a usable wash-out period of about 2–4 minutes. Spectral Doppler examinations of, for example, the pulmonary vein, that fail because of lack of signal strength, can be 'rescued' by the contrast examination, detecting signals that would be otherwise obscured by noise.

1.3.2.1 Enhancement studies with conventional imaging

In the initial studies which were carried out to obtain regulatory approval of ultrasound contrast agents, the sole indication was to salvage a nondiagnostic Doppler examination. These demonstrated the capacity of contrast agents to increase the technical success rate of Doppler assessments of aortic stenosis, mitral regurgitation and pulmonary venous flow, in which latter case it rose from 27 percent to 80 percent (22).

Echo enhancement caused by the agent may be considered in other ways too. For example, given a satisfactory transthoracic colour Doppler study, one use of the agent might be simply to enable a higher ultrasound frequency to be used, exploiting the agent to counter the higher tissue attenuation. In such a case, the contrast enhancement translates into higher spatial resolution (Figure 3). Alternatively, the colour system may be set to use fewer pulses per scan line (that is a lower ensemble length) while still achieving the same sensitivity to blood flow by means of the contrast enhancement. The agent will then provide the user with a higher frame rate.

With conventional greyscale imaging, enhancement might be seen in lumina of the ventricles or large vessels if the concentration of the bubbles is sufficiently high, as it is for perfluorocarbon gas agents such as Optison and Definity. The contrast is not, however, normally seen in the small vessels within the muscle of the myocardium itself. This is because the 10–25 dB of enhancement provided by the agent still leaves the blood echo some 10–20 dB below that of the echogenic tissue of the heart wall. In order to enhance the visible grey level, either higher concentrations of bubbles must be achieved or specific, new imaging strategies employed. A greater number of bubbles, however, inevitably leads to higher attenuation of the sound beam as it traverses the cavities, so perfusion imaging cannot be effective using conventional imaging (23). Thus new, bubble specific imaging methods are necessary.

1.3.3 II – Nonlinear backscatter: harmonic imaging

1.3.3.1 The need for bubble-specific imaging

In many of the potential applications of contrast agents, one might ask whether it is possible to continue to increase the amount of agents injected and obtain progressively stronger echoes from blood; to the point, for example, where the myocardium becomes visible on a greyscale image. Unfortunately, attenuation of the ultrasound beam by the agent in the cavity also increases with bubble concentration, with the result that shadowing occurs distal to the agent and the myocardium disappears altogether. Because of this limitation of the useable concentration of the agent, we are generally left with small enhancements in the myocardium echo that must be identified against the strong background echo from the solid tissue itself. X-ray angiography, which is faced with a similar problem after dye is injected into the bloodstream, deals with these 'clutter' components of the image by simple subtraction of a pre-injection image. What is left behind reveals flow in individual vessels or the 'blush' of perfusion at the tissue level. If, however, we subtract two consecutive ultrasound images of a solid organ, we get a third ultrasound image of the same organ, produced by the decorrelation of the speckle pattern between acquisitions. In order to show parenchymal enhancement due to the agent, speckle variance must first be reduced by filtering, with a consequent loss of spatial or temporal resolution. Even if the speckle problem could be overcome, subtraction would still be poorly suited to the dynamic and interactive nature of cardiac ultrasound imaging. In Doppler modes, the problem of the moving wall interference (the clutter) prevents the smaller echo from the blood itself being detected, as discussed in §1.1.3.

How then might contrast agents be used to improve the visibility of blood in moving vascular structures such as the myocardium? Clearly, a method that could identify the echo from the contrast agent and suppress the echo from solid tissue would provide both a real time 'subtraction' mode for contrast-enhanced B-mode imaging, and a means of suppressing Doppler clutter without the use of a velocity-dependent filter in spectral and colour modes. Nonlinear imaging aims to provide such a method, and hence the means for detection of flow in smaller vessels than is currently possible.

1.3.3.2 Harmonic imaging

Examining the behaviour of contrast-enhanced ultrasound studies reveals two important pieces of evidence. First, the size of the echo enhancement at very high dilution following a small peripheral injection (7 dB from as little as 0.01 ml/kg of Levovist, for example (24)) is much larger than would be expected from such sparse scatterers of this size in blood. Second, investigations of the acoustic characteristics of several agents (25) have demonstrated an approximately linear dependence of backscattered coefficient on numerical density of the agent at low concentrations, as expected, but a dependence of attenuation on ultrasound frequency different to that predicted by the Rayleigh law, which describes how the echogenicity of normal tissue changes with frequency. Instead, peaks exist which are dependent on both ultrasound frequency and the size of the microbubbles, suggestive of resonance phenomena. This important observation suggests that the bubbles *resonate* in the ultrasound field. As the ultrasound wave – which comprises alternate compressions and rarefactions – propagates over the bubbles, they experience a periodic change in their radius in sympathy with the oscillations of the incident sound. Like vibrations in other structures, these radial oscillations have a natural – or resonant – frequency of oscillation at which they will both absorb and scatter ultrasound with a peculiarly high efficiency. Considering the linear oscillation of a free bubble of air in water, we can use a simple theory (1) to predict the resonant frequency of radial oscillation of a bubble of 3 µm diameter, the median diameter of a typical transpulmonary microbubble agent. As Figure 20 shows, it is about 3 MHz,

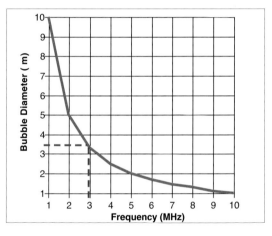

Fig. 20 Microbubbles resonate in a diagnostic ultrasound field. This graph shows that the resonant – or natural – frequency of oscillation of a bubble of air in an ultrasound field depends on its size. For a 3.5 µm diameter, the size needed for an intravenously injectable contrast agent, the resonant frequency is about 3 MHz.

approximately the centre frequency of ultrasound used in a typical echocardiography scan. This extraordinary – and fortunate – coincidence explains why ultrasound contrast agents are so efficient and can be administered in such small quantities. It also predicts that bubbles undergoing resonant oscillation in an ultrasound field can be induced to emit harmonics, the basis of harmonic imaging.

One consequence of this extraordinary coincidence is that bubbles undergoing resonant oscillation in an ultrasound field can be induced to nonlinear motion. It has long been recognised (26) that if bubbles are 'driven' by the ultrasound field at sufficiently high acoustic pressures, the oscillatory excursions of the bubble reach a point where the alternate expansions and contractions of the bubble's size are not equal. Lord Rayleigh, the originator of the theoretical understanding of sound upon which ultrasound imaging is based, was first led in 1917 to investigate this by his curiosity over the creaking noises that his teakettle made as the water came to the boil. The consequence of such nonlinear motion is

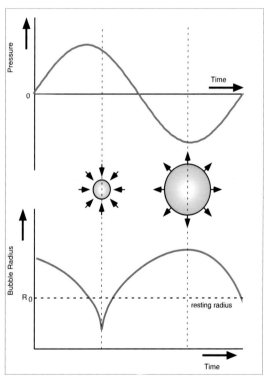

Fig. 21 Higher incident pressures induce nonlinear behaviour in a bubble. Asymmetric oscillation of a resonant bubble in an ultrasound field gives rise to an echo with even harmonics.

that the sound emitted by the bubble, and detected by the transducer, contains harmonics, just as the resonant strings of a musical instrument, if plucked too vigorously, will produce a 'harsh' timbre containing *overtones* (the musical term for harmonics). The origin of this phenomenon is the asymmetry which begins to affect resonant oscillation as the amplitude becomes large. As a bubble is compressed by the ultrasound pressure wave, it becomes stiffer and hence resists further reduction in its radius. Conversely, in the rarefaction phase of the ultrasound pulse, the bubble becomes less stiff, and, therefore, enlarges much more (Figure 21). Figure 22 shows the frequency spectrum of an echo produced by a microbubble contrast agent following a 3.75 MHz burst. The particular agent is Levovist, though many microbubble agents behave in a similar way. Ultrasound frequency is on the horizontal axis, with the relative amplitude on the vertical axis. A strong echo, at -13 dB with respect to the fundamental, is seen at twice the transmitted frequency, the second harmonic. Peaks in the echo spectrum at sub- and ultraharmonics are also seen. Here, then, is one potential method to distinguish bubbles from tissue: excite them so as to produce harmonics and detect these in preference to the fundamental echo from tissue. Key factors in the harmonic response of an agent, which varies from material to material, are the incident pressure of the ultrasound field, the frequency, as well as the size distribution of the bubbles and the mechanical properties of the bubble capsule. A stiff capsule, for example, will dampen the

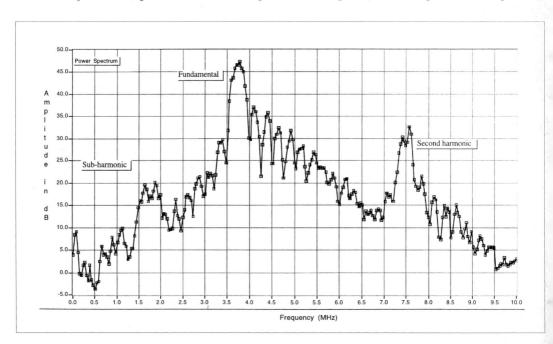

Fig. 22 Harmonic emission from Levovist. A sample of a contrast agent is insonated at 3.75 MHz and the echo analyzed for its frequency content. It is seen that most of the energy in the echo is at 3.75 MHz, but that there is a clear second peak in the spectrum at 7.5 MHz, as well as a third at 1.875 MHz. The second harmonic echo is only 13 dB less than that of the main, or fundamental echo. Harmonic imaging and Doppler aims to separate and process this signal alone. The smaller peak is the first subharmonic.

oscillations and attenuate the nonlinear response.

Harmonic B-mode imaging

A new real-time imaging and Doppler method based on this principle, called harmonic imaging (27), is now widely available on most modern echocardiography ultrasound scanners. In harmonic mode, the system transmits normally at one frequency, but when in harmonic mode is tuned to receive echoes preferentially at double that frequency, where the echoes from the bubbles lie. Typically, the transmit frequency lies between 1.5 and 3 MHz and the receive frequency is selected by means of a bandpass filter whose centre frequency is at the second harmonic between 3 and 6 MHz (Figure 23). Harmonic imaging uses the same array transducers as conventional imaging and for in most of today's ultrasound systems involves only software changes. Echoes from solid tissue, as well as red blood cells themselves, are suppressed. Real-time harmonic spectral Doppler and colour Doppler modes have also been implemented (sometimes experimentally) on a number of commercially available systems. Clearly, an exceptional transducer bandwidth is needed to operate over such a large range of frequencies. Fortunately much effort has been directed in recent years towards increasing the bandwidth of transducer arrays because of its significant bearing on conventional imaging performance, so harmonic imaging modes do not require the additional expense of dedicated transducers.

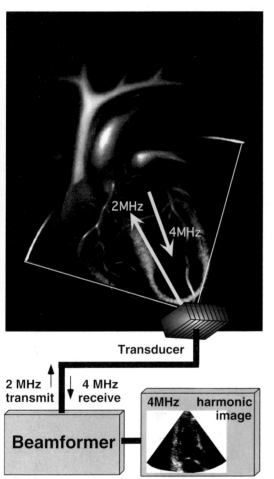

Fig. 23 The principle of harmonic imaging and Doppler. A conventional phased array is used, with the receiver tuned to double the transmitting frequency. The tissue and blood give an echo at the fundamental frequency, but the contrast agent undergoing nonlinear oscillation in the sound field emits the harmonic which is detected by the harmonic system.

Harmonic Doppler imaging

In harmonic images, the echo from tissue mimicking material is reduced – but not eliminated, reversing the contrast between the agent and its surrounding (Figure 24). The value of this effect is to increase the conspicuity of the agent when it is in blood vessels normally hidden by the strong echoes from tissue. In spectral Doppler, one would expect the suppression of the tissue echo to reduce the tissue motion 'thump' that is familiar to all echocardiographers. Figure 25 shows spectral Doppler applied to a region of the aorta in

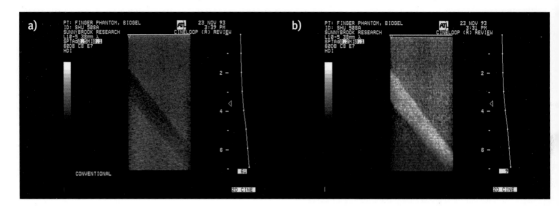

Fig. 24 Harmonic imaging. An vitro phantom shows a finger-like void in tissue equivalent material, filled with dilute contrast agent, barely visible in conventional mode (a). Harmonic imaging is seen to reverse the contrast between the microbubble agent and the surrounding material (b).

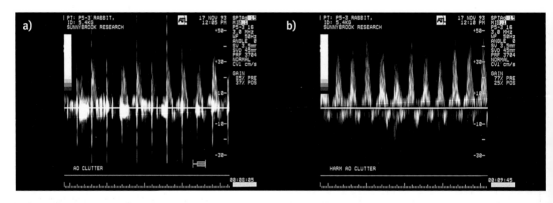

Fig. 25 Clutter rejection with harmonic spectral Doppler. (a) The abdominal aorta of an animal is examined with harmonic spectral Doppler. In conventional mode, clutter from the moving wall causes the familiar artifact which also obscures diastolic flow. (b) In harmonic mode, the clutter is almost completely suppressed, so that flow can be resolved. The settings of the filter and other relevant instrument parameters are identical.

which there is wall motion as well as blood flow within the sample volume. The conventional Doppler image of Figure 25 a shows the thump artifact due to clutter, which is almost completely absent in the harmonic Doppler image of Figure 25 b. All instrument settings, including the filters, are identical in these images; we have merely switched between modes. In vivo measurements from spectral Doppler show that the signal-to-clutter ratio is improved by a combination of harmonic imaging and the contrast agent by as much as 35 dB (28). Figure 26 shows harmonic colour images of an aorta, this time with flash artifact from respiratory motion. The harmonic image demonstrates the flow without the flash artifact. The potential application of this diagnostic method is to detect blood flow in small

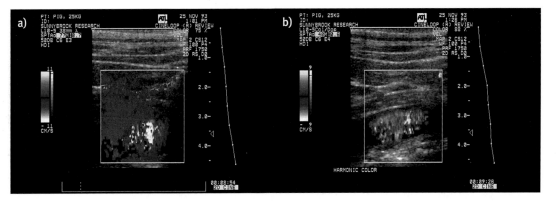

Fig. 26 Clutter rejection with harmonic colour Doppler. (a) Flow in the abdominal aorta is superimposed on respiratory motion, producing severe flash artifact. (b) In harmonic mode at the same point in the respiratory cycle, the flash artifact disappears. Flow from a smaller vessel (the cranial mesenteric artery) is visualised. All instrument settings are the same.

vessels surrounded by tissue which is moving: in the branches of the coronary arteries (29) or the myocardium itself (30), as well as in the parenchyma of abdominal organs (31).

Harmonic power Doppler imaging

In colour Doppler studies using a contrast agent, the effect of the arrival of the agent in a colour region of interest is often to produce 'blooming' of the colour image, whereby signals from major vascular targets spread out to occupy the entire region. Thus, although flow from smaller vessels might be detectable, the colour images can be swamped by artifactual flow signals. The origin of this artifact is the amplitude thresholding that governs most colour displays in conventional (or 'velocity') mode imaging. Increasing the backscattered signal power simply has the effect of displaying the velocity estimate, at full intensity, over a wider range of pixels around the detected location. A display in which the parameter mapped to colour is related directly to the backscattered signal power, on the other hand, has the advantage that such thresholding is unneccessary and that lower amplitude Doppler shifts, such as those which result from sidelobe interference, are displayed at a lower visual amplitude, rendering them less conspicuous. Echo enhanced flow signals, in contrast, will be displayed at a higher level. This is the basis of the power imaging map (also known as colour power angiography, or colour Doppler energy mapping). Power Doppler can help eliminate some other limitations of small vessel flow detection with colour Doppler. Low velocity detection requires lowering the Doppler pulse repetition frequency (PRF), which results in multiple aliasing and loss of directional resolution. A display method that does not use the velocity estimate is not prone to the aliasing artifact, and therefore allows the PRF to be lowered and hence increase the likelihood of detection of the lower velocity flow from smaller vessels.

Because it maps a parameter directly related to the acoustic quantity that is enhanced by the contrast agent, the power map is a natural choice for contrast enhanced colour Doppler studies. However, the advantages of the power map for contrast enhanced detection of small vessel flow are balanced by a potentially devas-

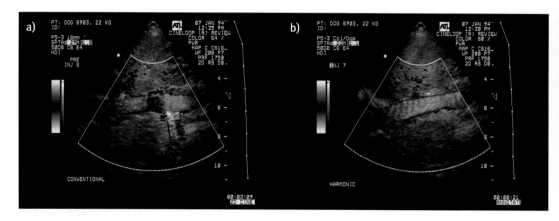

Fig. 27 Reduction of the flash artifact in harmonic power Doppler. The harmonic contrast method helps overcome one of the principal shortcomings of power Doppler, its increased susceptibility to tissue motion. (a) Aortic flow in power mode with flash artifact from cardiac motion of wall. (b) In harmonic mode at the same point in the cardiac cycle, the flash is largely suppressed. All instrument settings are the same.

tating shortcoming: its increased susceptibility to interference from clutter. Clutter is both detected more readily, because of the power mode's increased sensitivity, and displayed more prominently, because of the high intensity display of high amplitude signals. Furthermore, frame averaging has the additional effect of sustaining and blurring the flash over the cardiac cycle, so exacerbating its effect on the image. This is the reason that conventional power mode, while quite popular in radiological and peripheral vascular ultrasound imaging, has almost no role in echocardiography.

At the small expense of some sensitivity, amply compensated by the enhancement caused by the agent, harmonic mode effectively overcomes this clutter problem (Figure 27). Combining the harmonic method with power Doppler produces an especially effective tool for the detection of flow in the small vessels of the organs of the abdomen which may be moving with cardiac pulsation or respiration. In a study in which flow imaged on contrast enhanced power harmonic images was compared with histologically sized arterioles in the corresponding regions of the renal cortex (24), it was concluded that the method is capable of demonstrating flow in vessels of less than 40μm diameter; about ten times smaller than the corresponding imaging resolution limit, even as the organ was moving with normal respiration. Recent studies of this power mode method in the heart (32) show that flow can be imaged in the myocardium with an agent such as Levovist (33).

1.3.3.3 The impact of harmonic imaging

Harmonic imaging succeeds in identifying microbubble contrast agent in the tissue vasculature by means of its echo 'signature'. In doing so it helps tackle some old problems in ultrasound, such as the rejection of the tissue echo in Doppler modes designed to image moving blood, and creating a 'subtraction' mode without sacrificing the real time nature of the examination. Figure 28 summarises graphically the effect of contrast agents and harmonic detection on the Doppler process. In conventional Doppler, the signal from blood is larger

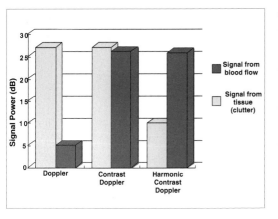

Fig. 28 Quantifying the impact of harmonic Doppler. Clutter and spectral Doppler signal levels measured in conventional, contrast enhanced, and harmonic contrast enhanced modes.

than the clutter signal from tissue. In contrast enhanced Doppler, the signal from blood is raised, sometimes to near that of tissue. With harmonic mode, the signal from blood is raised but that from the tissue reduced, so reversing the contrast between tissue and blood. Another way of looking at the harmonic method is that, because of its greater sensitivity to small quantities of agent, a given level of enhancement due to a bolus will last longer (Figure 29). This is the reason that a number of investigators have found that cardiac contrast imaging in any mode is generally more effective with the harmonic method (29, 30). Harmonic imaging has been shown to render possible the detection of microvessels containing contrast agents even in the presence of highly echogenic tissue, such as the liver (31) and myocardium (34).

Harmonic imaging demands exceptional performance from the transducer array and system beamformer. Its implementation forces implicit compromises between, for example, image resolution and rejection of the non-contrast agent echo. It places unusual demands on the bandwidth performance of transducers, as well as the flexibility of the architecture of the imaging system. The ease with which it has been developed on modern instruments, however,

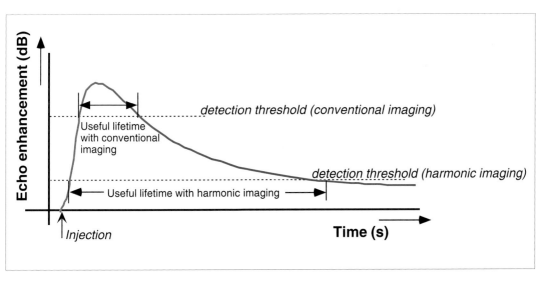

Fig. 29 The improved sensitivity of the harmonic method translates into increased useful imaging time from a contrast agent bolus. Time-enhancement curve caused by circulation of contrast agent bolus shows how harmonic imaging, by reducing the detection threshold, increases the imaging lifetime of the agent.

Harmonic imaging modalities

Method	Usual Format	Application
Harmonic B-mode	Greyscale display of harmonic echoes	LVO; myocardial perfusion (offline subtraction necessary)
Harmonic spectral Doppler	Spectral Doppler with tissue motion suppression	Coronary flow reserve; pulmonary vein Doppler enhancement
Harmonic colour Doppler	Colour Doppler with tissue suppression, conventional B-mode background	Coronary vessel imaging
Harmonic power Doppler	Power Doppler with tissue motion suppression, conventional B-mode background	LVO; myocardial perfusion

reflects this flexibility and augurs well for the future of the method. More significantly, contrast agents are now being developed specifically with nonlinear response as a design criterion. Entirely new agents present opportunities for entirely new detection strategies (17). Our laboratory measurements show that some new contrast agents are capable of creating an echo with more energy in the second harmonic than at the fundamental: that is, they are more efficient in harmonic than conventional mode. With such agents, nonlinear imaging is the preferred clinical method for their detection.

1.3.3.4 Tissue harmonic imaging

In second harmonic imaging, an ultrasound scanner transmits at one frequency and receives at double this frequency. The resulting improved detection of the microbubble echo is due to the peculiar behaviour of a gas bubble in an ultrasound field. However, any source of a received signal at the harmonic frequency which does not come from the bubble, will clearly reduce the efficacy of this method.

Such unwanted signals can come from non-linearities in the transducer or its associated electronics, and these must be tackled effectively in a good harmonic imaging system. However, tissue itself can produce harmonics which will be received by the transducer. They are developed as a wave propagates through tissue. Again, this is due to an asymmetry: this time the fact that sound travels slightly faster through tissue during the compressional part of the cycle (where it is denser and hence more stiff) than during the rarefactional part. Although this effect is very small, it is sufficient to produce substantial harmonic components in the transmitted wave by the time it reaches deep tissue, so that when it is scattered by a linear target such as the myocardium, there is a harmonic component in the echo, which is detected by the scanner along with the harmonic echo from the bubble (35). This is the reason that solid tissue is not completely dark in a typical harmonic image. The effect is to reduce the contrast between the bubble and tissue, rendering the problem of detecting perfusion in the myocardium more difficult.

Tissue harmonics, though a foe to contrast imaging, are not necessarily a bad thing. In fact, an image formed from tissue harmonics without the presence of contrast agents has some properties which recommend it over conventional imaging. These follow from the fact that tissue harmonics are developed as the beam penetrates tissue, in contrast to the conventional beam, which is generated at the transducer surface (36). Artifacts which accrue

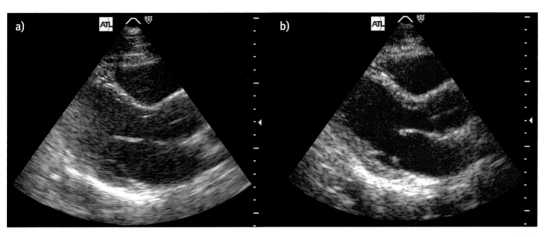

Fig. 30 Tissue harmonic imaging of the heart. Note that in comparison to the fundamental image (a), the tissue harmonic image (b) has a reduced level of artifacts associated with reverberation and sidelobe interference.

from the first few centimetres of tissue, such as reverberations, are reduced by using tissue harmonic imaging. Sidelobe and other low-level interference is also suppressed, making tissue harmonic imaging the routine modality of choice for many echocardiographers (Figure 30).

Potential origin of echoes at harmonic frequency

- Nonlinear scattering from bubbles
- Nonlinear propagation of echoes from solid tissue
- Inadvertent transmission of harmonics by non-linearities in transmitter or transducer
- Inadvertent production of harmonics by non-linearities in receiver or transducer
- Deliberate transmission at second harmonic frequency to improve bandwidth of image

For contrast studies, the tissue harmonic limits the visibilty of bubbles within tissue in a B-mode harmonic image and therefore can be considered an artifact. In contemplating how to reduce it, it is instructive to bear in mind differences between harmonics produced by tissue propagation and by bubble echoes. First, tissue harmonics require a high peak pressure, so are only evident at high MI. Reducing the MI leaves only the bubble harmonics. Second, tissue harmonics become greater at greater depths, whereas harmonics from bubbles are depth independent. Finally, harmonics from tissue at high MI are continuous and sustained, whereas those from bubbles are transient in nature as the bubble disrupts.

1.3.3.5 Pulse inversion imaging

The method we have described above for harmonic imaging imposes some fundamental limitations on the imaging process which restrict its clinical potential in organ imaging. First, in order to ensure that the higher frequencies are due only to harmonics emitted by the bubbles, the transmitter must be restricted to a band of frequencies around the fundamental (Figure 31 a). Similarly, the received band of frequencies must be restricted to those lying around the second harmonic. If these two regions overlap (Figure 31 b), the result will be that the harmonic filter will receive echoes

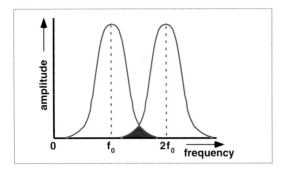

Fig. 31 a) The compromises forced by harmonic imaging: In harmonic imaging, the transmitted frequencies must be restricted to a band around the fundamental, and the receive frequencies must be limited to a band around the second harmonic. This limits resolution.

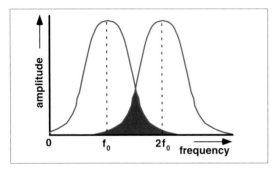

Fig. 31 b) If the transmit and receive bandwidths are increased to improve resolution, some fundamental echoes from tissue will overlap the receive bandwidth and will be detected, reducing contrast between agent and tissue.

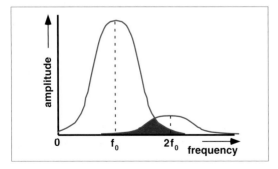

Fig. 31 c) When the harmonic echoes are weak, due to low agent concentration and/or low incident pulse intensity, this overlap will be especially large, and the harmonic signal may be largely composed of tissue echoes.

from ordinary tissue, thus reducing the contrast between the agent and tissue. However, restricting the receive bandwidth degrades the resolution of the resulting image, thus framing a fundamental compromise in harmonic imaging between contrast and resolution. For optimal detection of bubbles in the microvasculature, this compromise must favour contrast, so that the most sensitive harmonic images are generally of low quality. In other applications where the bubble echo has a higher intensity, such as in the ventricular cavities, higher bandwidths can be tolerated. A further drawback of the filtering approach to harmonic imaging is illustrated in Figure 31 c. There it can be seen that if the received echo is weak, the overlapping region between the transmit and received frequencies becomes large relative to the whole received signal. This means that contrast in the harmonic image is dependent on how strong the echo is from the bubbles, which is determined by the concentration of bubbles and the intensity of the incident ultrasound pulse. In practice, this dictates that scanning in harmonic mode must be performed with a high mechanical index, that is, using the maximum transmit power of the system. This results in the transient and irreversible disruption of the bubbles (37). Consequently, as the bubbles enter the scan plane of a real-time ultrasound image, they provide an echo but then disappear. Thus vessels that lie within the scan plane are not visualised as tubular structures in a typical harmonic image, but instead have a punctate appearance.

Principle of pulse inversion
Pulse inversion imaging overcomes the conflict between the requirements of contrast and resolution in harmonic imaging and provides greater sensitivity, thus allowing low incident

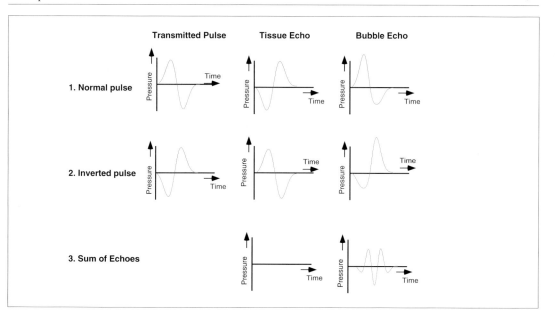

Fig. 32 Principle of Pulse Inversion Imaging. A pulse of sound is transmitted into the body and echoes are received from agent and tissue. A second pulse, which is an inverted copy of the first pulse, is then transmitted in the same direction and the two echoes are summed. Linear echoes from tissue will be inverted copies of each other and will cancel to zero. The microbubble echoes are distorted copies of each other, and the nonlinear components of these echoes will reinforce each other when summed, producing a strong harmonic signal.

power, nondestructive, continuous imaging of microbubbles in an organ such as the liver. The method also relies on the asymmetric oscillation of an ultrasound bubble in an acoustic field, but detects all nonlinear (or, 'even') components of the echo, over the entire bandwidth of the transducer. In pulse inversion imaging, two pulses are sent in rapid succession into the tissue. The second pulse is a mirror image of the first (Figure 32). That is, it has undergone a 180° phase change. The scanner detects the echo from these two successive pulses and forms their sum. For ordinary tissue, which behaves in a linear manner, the sum of two inverted pulses is simply zero. For an echo with nonlinear components, such as that from a bubble, on the other hand, the echoes produced from these two pulses will not be simple mirror images of each other, because of the asymmetric behaviour of the bubble radius with time. The result is that the sum of these two echoes is not zero. Thus, a signal is detected from a bubble but not from tissue. It can be shown by mathematical analysis that this summed echo contains the nonlinear 'even' harmonic components of the signal, including the second harmonic (38).

One advantage of pulse inversion over the filter approach to detect harmonics from bubbles is that it no longer suffers from the restriction of bandwidth. The full frequency range of sound emitted from the transducer can be detected in this way, and a full bandwidth, that is high resolution, image of the nonlinear echoes from bubbles may be formed in real time. The price paid, using current technology, is a reduction of the effective frame rate by a factor of two.

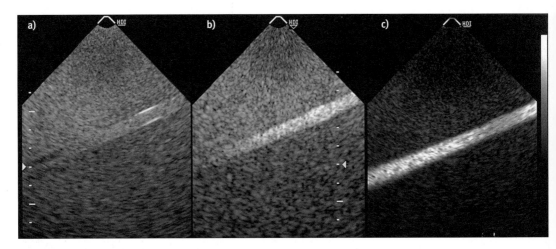

Fig. 33 Demonstration of pulse inversion imaging. In vitro images of a vessel phantom containing stationary Optison surrounded by tissue equivalent material (biogel and graphite). a) Conventional image, MI = 0.2. b) Harmonic imaging, MI = 0.2, provides improved contrast between agent and tissue. c) Pulse inversion imaging, MI = 0.2. By suppressing linear echoes from stationary tissue, pulse inversion imaging provides better contrast between agent and tissue than both conventional and harmonic imaging.

One application for this advantage is in tissue imaging without contrast agents. In conventional imaging, reverberation, phase aberration and sidelobe artifacts caused by the linear sound beam can reduce image contrast, especially in hypoechoic structures such as the ventricular cavities. Tissue harmonic imaging can reduce these artifacts and improve image contrast, but with a somewhat degraded resolution. Figure 37 illustrates how pulse inversion imaging provides better suppression of linear echoes than harmonic imaging and is effective over the full bandwidth of the transducer, showing improvement of image resolution over harmonic mode.

Because this detection method is a more efficient means of isolating the bubble echo, weaker echoes from bubbles insonated at low, nondestructive intensities, can be detected. Figure 33 shows a dramatic improvement in contrast sensitivity obtained over both fundamental and harmonic modes by pulse inversion imaging in a phantom. For LVO, pulse inversion imaging provides improved resolution of the endocardium (Figure 34). At high MI, bubbles are disrupted and their contents

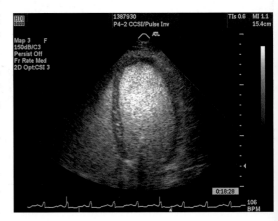

Fig. 34 Pulse inversion imaging with Levovist showing LV opacification. Notice that perforating branches of the coronary vessels are visible. *Courtesy Eric Yu, University of Toronto, Canada*

Principles and Instrumentation

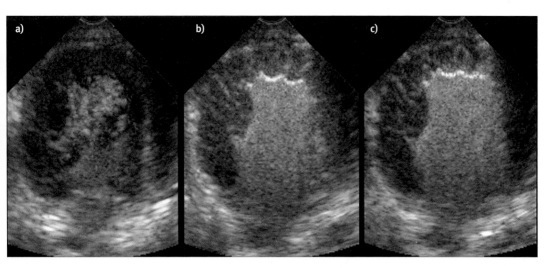

Fig. 35 Pulse inversion imaging showing coronary vessels using Levovist at two frames per heart beat. (a) Agent enters cavity. (b) Perfusion, 6 seconds later. (c) One second later, vessels are seen entering the myocardium.

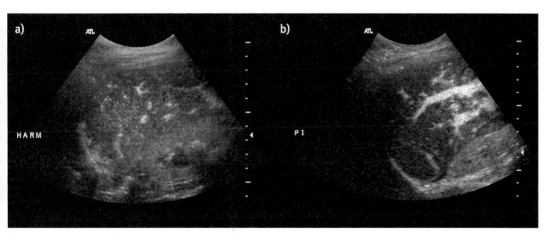

Fig. 36 The appearance of blood vessels in harmonic and pulse inversion imaging in a liver.
In a harmonic image of a liver following an injection of Optison, large vessels have a punctate appearance as the high MI ultrasound disrupts the bubbles as they enter the scan plane (a). In the pulse inversion image of the same liver, a lower MI can be used so that continuous vessels are now seen. Improved resolution of pulse inversion imaging demonstrates 4th order branches of the portal vein (b).

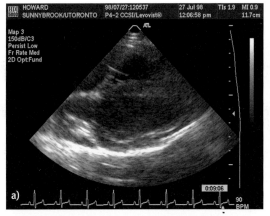

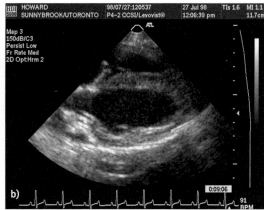

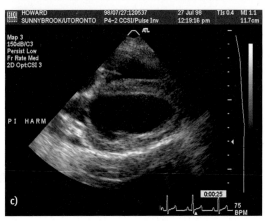

Fig. 37 Tissue harmonic imaging. In conventional image (a), reverberation, phase aberration and sidelobe artifacts degrade depiction of cavity borders. Tissue harmonic image (b) shows reduced artifacts, but with a somewhat degraded resolution. Pulse inversion image (c) gives better suppression of artifacts than harmonic imaging and uses full bandwidth of the transducer, thus improving resolution.

dispersed following insonation (see §1.3.4). Perforating coronary vessels, however, which have a sufficiently high flow velocity to refill between frames, become visible on pulse inversion images with Levovist (Figure 34–35). In the liver, low MI imaging allows long lengths of vessels to become visible. Figure 36 compares the appearance of large hepatic vessels imaged in harmonic and pulse inversion modes following a peripheral venous injection of Optison. The high MI harmonic image (Figure 36 a) shows the punctate appearance of vessels in which the agent is destroyed; the lower MI pulse inversion image (Figure 36 b) shows fourth order branches of the portal vein imaged with great clarity. Finally, because of its extended bandwidth, pulse inversion imaging is an ideal method to use for high MI tissue harmonic imaging. Figure 37 compares the fundamental (Figure 37 a), harmonic (Figure 37 b) and pulse inversion images (Figure 37 c) of the same view. Note that artifact suppression is achieved in both the harmonic and pulse inversion images, but that the resolution of the pulse inversion image is superior.

1.3.3.6 Power pulse inversion imaging

In spite of the improvements offered by pulse inversion over harmonic imaging for suppressing stationary tissue, the method is somewhat sensitive to echoes from moving tissue. This is because movement of tissue causes linear

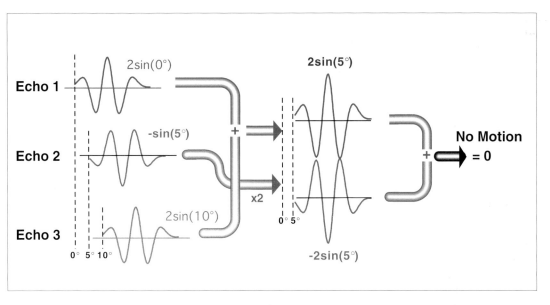

Fig. 38 The principle of pulse inversion Doppler (also known as *power pulse inversion*). The method is similar to pulse inversion imaging, except that a sequence of more than two pulses are transmitted with alternating phase. The echoes from successive pulses are recombined in a way that eliminates the effect of steady displacement of the target due to tissue motion. The method allows suppression of moving tissue without the need to disrupt the bubble, hence achieving real time, low MI imaging. The example shown here of three pulses illustrates a principle that can be applied to arbitrarily long ensembles of pulses, improving bubble-to-tissue sensitivity.

echoes to change slightly between pulses, so that they do not cancel perfectly. Furthermore, at high MI, nonlinear propagation also causes harmonic echoes to appear in pulse inversion images, even from linear scattering structures such as solid tissue. While tissue motion artifacts can be minimised by using a short pulse repetition interval, nonlinear tissue echoes can mask the echoes from bubbles, reducing the efficacy of microbubble contrast, especially in interval delay imaging when a high MI is used. A recent development seeks to address these problems by means of a generalisation of the pulse inversion method, called pulse inversion Doppler (38). This technique – which is also known as *power pulse inversion* imaging – combines the nonlinear detection performance of pulse inversion imaging with the motion discrimination capabilities of power Doppler. Multiple transmit pulses of alternating polarity are used and Doppler signal processing techniques are applied to distinguish between bubble echoes and echoes from moving tissue and/or tissue harmonics, as desired by the operator. In a typical configuration, the echoes from a train of pulses are combined in such a way that signals from moving tissue – which pose a problem to pulse inversion imaging – are eliminated (Figure 38). This method offers improvements in the agent to tissue contrast and signal to noise performance, though at the cost of a somewhat reduced framerate. The most dramatic manifestation of this method's ability to detect very weak harmonic echoes has been its first demonstration of real-time perfusion imaging of the myocardium (39)

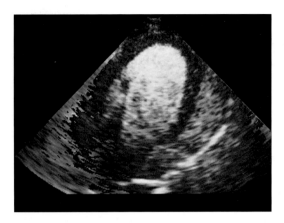

Fig. 39 Pulse inversion Doppler (also known as 'power pulse inversion') showing real-time myocardial perfusion. The contrast agent is Optison, the mechanical index is 0.15, the frame rate is 15 Hz.

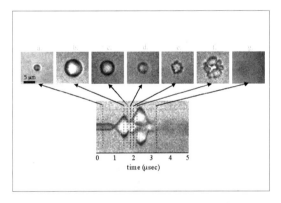

Fig. 40 Fragmentation of contrast agent observed with a high-speed camera. The frame images (a–g) are captured over 50 nanoseconds. The streak image (similar to an M-mode) shows the variations in bubble diameter with a temporal resolution of 10 nanoseconds. The bubble is insonified with 2.4 MHz ultrasound with a peak negative pressure of 1.1 MPa (MI~0.7). (a) The bubble is initially 3 μm in diameter. (b) The first large expansion. (c–d) The bubble fragments during compression after the first expansion. (e–f) Fragments are seen during expansion. Resulting bubble fragments are not seen after insonation, because they are either fully dissolved or below the optical resolution.
Courtesy of James Chomas, Paul Dayton, Kathy Ferrara, University of California, Davis CA, USA

(Figure 39). By lowering the MI to 0.1 or less, bubbles undergo stable, nonlinear oscillation, emitting continuous harmonic signals. Because of the low MI, very few bubbles are disrupted, so that imaging can take place at real-time rates. Because sustained, stable nonlinear oscillation is required for this method, perfluorocarbon gas bubbles work best.

1.3.4 III - Transient disruption: intermittent imaging

As the incident pressure to which a resonating bubble is exposed increases, so its oscillation becomes more wild, with radius increasing in some bubbles by a factor of five or more during the rarefaction phase of the incident sound. Just as a resonating violin string, if bowed overzealously, will break, so a microbubble, if driven by intense ultrasound, will suffer irreversible disruption of its shell. A physical picture of precisely what happens to a disrupted bubble is only now emerging from high speed video studies (Figure 40). It is certain, however, that the bubble disappears as an acoustic scatterer (not instantly, but over a period of time determined by the bubble composition), and that as it does so it emits a strong, brief nonlinear echo. It is this echo whose detection is the basis of intermittent myocardial perfusion imaging with ultrasound contrast agents.

1.3.4.1 Triggered imaging

It was discovered during the early days of harmonic imaging that by pressing the 'freeze' button on a scanner for a few moments, and hence interrupting the acquisition of ultrasound images during a contrast study, it is possible to increase the effectiveness of a contrast agent. So dramatic is this effect that it can raise

Principles and Instrumentation

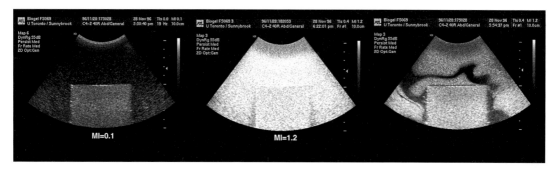

Fig. 41 Bubble disruption demonstrated in a laboratory phantom. a) Bubbles are suspended in a water bath containing a block of tissue mimicking material. b) The block is scanned at high mechanical index using a linear array scanner. A bright echo is seen from the bubbles as they experience high peak pressure insonation. c) An image taken a moment later reveals a swirl of echo-free fluid, corresponding to the scanplane which no longer bears intact bubbles. This explains the apical 'swirl' seen in many LVO studies at high MI.

the visibility of a contrast agent in the myocardial circulation to the point that it can be seen on a harmonic B-mode image, above the echo level of the normal heart muscle (40). This is a consequence of the ability of the ultrasound field, if its peak pressure is sufficiently high, to disrupt a bubble's shell and hence destroy it (37, 41) A phantom study illustrating this effect is shown in Figure 41. As the bubble is disrupted, it releases energy, so creating a strong, transient echo, which is rich in harmonics. This process is sometimes misleadingly referred to as 'stimulated acoustic emission'. The fact that this echo is transient in nature can be exploited for its detection. The first, and simplest method, is to subtract from a disruption image a baseline image obtained either before or (more usefully) immediately after insonation. The residual echoes can then be attributed to the bubbles which were disrupted by the imaging process. Such a method requires offline processing of stored ultrasound images, together with software which can align the ultrasound images before subtraction. Chapter 4 contains more discussion and examples of this technique. A more effective method is to compare the echoes from two or more consecutive high intensity pulses, separated by a fraction of a millisecond. This is the principle of intermittent harmonic power Doppler.

1.3.4.2 Intermittent harmonic power Doppler

Power Doppler imaging (also known as *colour power angio,* or *energy imaging*) is a technique designed to detect the motion of blood or of tissue. It works by a simple, pulse-to-pulse subtraction method (42), in which two or more pulses are sent successively along each scan line of the image. Pairs of received echo trains are compared for each line: if they are identical, nothing is displayed, but if there is a change (due to motion of the tissue between pulses), a colour is displayed whose saturation is related to the amplitude of the echo that has changed. This method, though not designed for the detection of bubble disruption, is ideally suited for high MI 'destruction' imaging. The first pulse receives an echo from the bubble, the second receives none, so the comparison yields a strong signal. In a sense, power Doppler may be thought of as a line-by-line

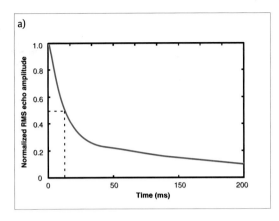 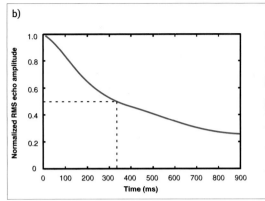

Fig. 42 Air bubbles disrupt more rapidly than do perfluorocarbon bubbles under high mechanical index insonation. In this experiment, bubbles from an air agent (a) and a perfluoropropane agent (b) are insonated under identical conditions. The half-life of the air bubble is approximately 20 ms, while the perfluropropane bubble is still providing an echo after 0.5 sec. The rapid response of the air agents at high MI is a strong advantage when they are imaged using intermittent harmonic power Doppler.

subtraction procedure on the radiofrequency echo detected by the transducer.

A crucial question is how long one needs to wait between pulses. If the two pulses are too close together in time, the bubble's gaseous contents, which are dispersed after disruption of the shell by a process of diffusion and fragmentation, will still be able to provide an echo, so reducing the effectiveness of the detection. If the two pulses are too far apart in time, the solid tissue of the myocardium will have moved, so that the detection process will show them as well. Of course, the amplitude of the echo from a block of muscle is much stronger than that from a micron-sized bubble within it, so this signal will mask that from the bubble. There are two solutions. First, by using harmonic detection, some – but not all – of the moving tissue 'clutter' can be rejected. Second, a bubble can be designed to disrupt quickly so that rapid (that is, high pulse repetition frequency (PRF)) imaging may be used. Such a bubble will have a gas content that is highly diffusible and soluble in blood. In this respect, air is perfect. Diffusion of air after acoustic disruption is about 40 times faster than such diffusion of a perfluorocarbon gas from a similar bubble (37), so that air based agents such as Levovist are easiest to image in this mode (Figure 42). For perfluorocarbon bubbles, longer insonation periods are necessary, but by using multiple pulses for each line (4–8 is typical) and careful filter design, very effective perfusion imaging can be achieved with these agents too. It is upon such considerations that the machine settings for perfusion imaging recommended in Chapter 3 are based.

Blood flow velocities in the vessels of the myocardium are very low, so that as soon as high MI imaging is commenced, bubbles are disrupted before they have time to refill the microvessels. Pausing the imaging process between acquisitions allows new agent to wash in and fill the vascular bed. The next imaging

Three methods for perfusion imaging

MI	Mode	Technique	Framerate (typical)
High	Harmonic B-mode or pulse inversion imaging	Intermittent imaging Offline subtraction of pre-contrast image	1/5 Hz
High	Harmonic power Doppler	Intermittent imaging Record first frame after disruption	1/5 Hz
Low	Power pulse inversion	Nondestructive, real-time imaging	16 Hz

pulse results in a strong echo, which is substantially stronger than the normal echo from the agent, and causes further destruction of the bubbles. This imaging strategy is sometimes referred to as 'intermittent' or 'transient' imaging. We (32) and others (30) have found that with harmonic imaging, this single acquisition imaging gives even more contrast. By combining intermittent harmonic imaging with power Doppler, one can assemble the most sensitive imaging mode so far available for contrast agents, with which have been demonstrated the first Doppler images of myocardial perfusion (32, 33). It is now commonplace to image a single frame over one, two, or up to eight heartbeats (Figure 43), so as to follow the time for the agent to refill the smallest vessels of the myocardium, into which the blood flows at only about 1 mm/s. Chapter 4 explores the opportunities for quantitation that this presents.

1.3.5 Summary

There are three regimes of behaviour of bubbles in an acoustic field, which depend on the intensity of the transmitted ultrasound beam. In practice, this intensity is best monitored by means of the mechanical index (MI) displayed by the scanner. At low MI, the bubbles act as simple, but powerful echo enhancers. This regime is most useful for spectral Doppler enhancement of, for example, pulmonary venous flow signals. At slightly higher intensities (the bottom of the range of those used diagnostically), the bubbles emit harmonics as they undergo nonlinear oscillation. These harmonics can be detected by harmonic and pulse inversion imaging, and form the basis of B-mode imaging for left ventricular opacification. By using the newer, more sensitive techniques such as power pulse

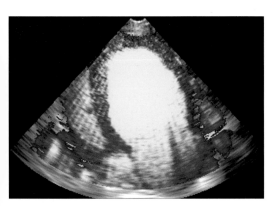

Fig. 43 Harmonic power Doppler image of myocardial perfusion, made using a trigger internal of four heartbeats.

inversion imaging, these echoes from bubbles can be separated from those due to tissue to give us real-time perfusion imaging of the myocardium. Finally, at the highest intensity setting of the machine used in routine scanning, the bubbles are disrupted, emitting a strong, transient echo. Detecting this echo with harmonic power Doppler remains the most sensitive means we have to image bubbles in very low concentration, but it comes at the price of destroying the bubble. Because of the long reperfusion periods of myocardial flow, intermittent imaging at framerates as low as one frame per eight heartbeats is then necessary.

1.4 Safety considerations

Contrast echocardiography exposes patients to ultrasound in a way that is identical to that of a normal echocardiography examination. Yet the use of ultrasound pulses to disrupt bubbles which sit in microscopic vessels raises some new questions about the potential for hazard. When a bubble produces the brief echo which is associated with its disruption, it releases energy which it has stored during its exposure to the ultrasound field. Can this energy damage the surrounding tissue? At higher exposure levels, ultrasound is known to produce bioeffects in tissue, the thresholds for which have been studied extensively. Do these thresholds change when bubbles are present in the vasculature? Whereas the safety of ultrasound contrast agents as drugs has been established to the satisfaction of the most stringent requirements of the regulating authorities in a number of countries, it is probably fair to say that there is much left to learn about the interaction between ultrasound and tissue when bubbles are present.

The most extreme of these interactions is known as cavitation. *Cavitation* refers to the formation, growth and collapse of a gas cavity in fluid as a result of ultrasound exposure. It has been studied extensively prior to the development of microbubble contrast agents (43). In fact, most of the mathematical models used to describe contrast microbubbles were originally developed to model cavitation (44–46). When sound waves of sufficient intensity travel through a fluid, the rarefactional half-cycle of the sound wave can actually tear the fluid apart, creating spherical cavities within the fluid. The subsequent rapid collapse of these cavities during the compressional half cycle of the sound wave can focus large amounts of energy into a very small volume, raising the temperature at the centre of the collapse to thousands of degrees Kelvin, forming free radicals, and even emitting electromagnetic radiation (sonoluminescence) (44–46).

The concern over potential cavitation-induced bioeffects in diagnostic ultrasound has lead to the development of several indices to describe the relative likelihood of cavitation from clinical instruments, of which the Mechanical Index described in §1.2.1.1 is now widely displayed on the monitors of most clinical ultrasound systems. With exception of one study which showed cavitation-induced hemorrhage in a mouse lung exposed under conditions that differ substantially from those found clinically (47), no evidence of bioeffects from conventional imaging at these levels have been reported. A number of experienced groups have carried out experiments to assess whether the presence of contrast microbubbles can act as cavitation seeds, potentiating cavitation-induced bioeffects (48–54). While much of this work has shown that adding contrast agents to blood increased cavitation effects (e.g. peroxide formation, acoustic emissions) and related bioeffects (e.g. hemolysis, platelet lysis), all significant bioeffects occurred with either very high agent concentration, sound pulse duration or MI, or with hematocrit well below the physiological range. In experiments in which clinically relevant values of these parameters were used (agent concentration <0.2 percent, pulse duration <2 µs, MI<1.9, hematocrit 40–45 percent), no significant bioeffects have been reported to date (49, 55).

1.5 New developments in contrast imaging

1.5.1 Tissue specific bubbles

As manufacturers of the agents gain more control over the rather difficult process of producing stable microbubbles, the possibilities to tailor their behaviour in the body increase. One of the most significant efforts is to target agents to specific sites in the body. Agents have been developed that adhere to thrombus, for example (56). Initial in vitro studies show a 6 dB enhancement of clot by the agent when imaged with intravascular ultrasound (57). The potential for such materials is clear, though the question remains as to the proportion of injected material that will reach the desired target and the dose needed to attain the desired contrast.

This dose can be minimised if the targeted agent itself contains gas. As described above, agents that are phagocytosed and remain intact in the Kupffer cells offer the prospect of a new kind of ultrasound liver imaging. However, until recently only particles have successfully performed this function. Recently a gas based agent (SHU 563, Schering AG, Berlin) has been developed which comprises a polymer particle with a gas filled interior. The mean particle size is approximately 1µm and the agent acts as an efficient ultrasound contrast agent in its blood pool phase, with extremely strong harmonic emission (55). After 15–20 minutes the agent is taken up, largely intact, into the reticuloendothelial system. When imaged with colour Doppler at high peak pressures, the bubbles are disrupted in the liver. The large change in signal level between two consecutive pulses is interpreted by the Doppler system as a random change in phase, and a random Doppler shift is assigned to this strong signal. The result is that the liver, though stationary, can be imaged with colour Doppler. Defects in the Kupffer cells brought about by, for example, a cancer, show as an absence of these Doppler signals. The method is so sensitive that we have shown that individual bubbles can be detected in this way; extremely low doses (3 µl/kg, for example) are all that is necessary. Using this technique, an isoechoic cancer of a diameter less than 2 mm has been imaged in an animal liver (17). This example of tissue-specific imaging using specially a designed contrast agent is likely to represent just the beginning of a completely new approach to the use of diagnostic ultrasound.

1.5.2 Bubbles for therapy

Future development of targeted agents can yield even more exciting prospects. By combining the targeting of an agent with the ability of diagnostic ultrasound to disrupt bubbles in a selected region in the body, a new method of drug delivery might become possible (58). Drugs could be delivered so that they attain toxic levels only in desired volumes of tissue.

Growth factors that enhance revascularisation may be potentiated by bubble-bound delivery and insonation over ischemic regions of tissue. Genetic material itself might be transported within a microbubble into a cell and released by acoustic means (59, 60).

1.6 Summary

Unlike contrast agents for other imaging modalities, microbubbles are modified by the process used to image them. Understanding the behaviour of bubbles while exposed to an ultrasound imaging beam is the key to performing an effective contrast echocardiography examination. The appropriate choice of a contrast specific imaging method is based on the behaviour of the agent and the requirements of the examination. The Mechanical Index (MI) is the major determinant of the response of contrast bubbles to ultrasound. Low MI harmonic and pulse inversion imaging offer real-time B-mode methods for left ventricular opacification. Harmonic spectral and colour Doppler may be used to suppress tissue motion in flow studies of coronary vessels. High MI harmonic power Doppler is ideally suited to intermittent imaging of myocardial perfusion with contrast agents, while power pulse inversion imaging at very low MI allows real-time visualisation of myocardial perfusion using perfluorocarbon agents.

1.7 References

1. Ophir J, Parker KJ. Contrast agents in diagnostic ultrasound. Ultrasound Med Biol 1989; 15:319–33.

2. Gramiak R, Shah PM. Echocardiography of the aortic root. Invest Radiol 1968; 3:356–366.

3. Ziskin MC, Bonakdapour A, Weinstein DP, Lynch PR. Contrast agents for diagnostic ultrasound. Invest Radiol 1972; 6:500–505.

4. Kremkau FW, Carstensen EL. Ultrasonic detection of cavitation at catheter tips. Am J Roentgenol 1968; 3:159–167.

5. Kerber RE, Kioschos JM, Lauer RM. Use of an ultrasonic contrast method in the diagnosis of valvular regurgitation and intracardiac shunts. Am J Cardiol 1974; 34:722–727.

6. Reid CL, Kawanishi DT, McKay CR. Accuracy of evaluation of the presence and severity of aortic and mitral regurgitation by contrast 2-dimensional echocardiography. Am J Cardiol 1983; 52:519–524.

7. Sahn DJ, Valdex-Cruz LM. Ultrasonic contrast studies for the detection of cardiac shunts. J Am Coll Cardiol 1984; 3: 978-985.

8. Roelandt J. Contrast echocardiography. Ultrasound Med Biol 1982; 8:471.

9. Carroll BA, Turner RJ, Tickner EG, Boyle DB, Young SW. Gelatin encapsulated nitrogen microbubbles as ultrasonic contrast agents. Invest Radiol 1980; 15:260–266.

10. Feinstein SB, Shah PM, Bing RJ, et al. Microbubble dynamics visualised in the intact capillary circulation. J Am CollCardiol 1984; 4:595–600.

11. Schlief R. Echo enhancement: agents and techniques – basic principles. Adv Echo-Contrast 1994; 4:5–19.

12. Fritzsch T, Schartl M, Siegert J. Preclinical and clinical results with an ultrasonic contrast agent. Invest Radiol 1988; 23:5.

13. Goldberg BB, Liu JB, Burns PN, Merton DA, Forsberg F. Galactose-based intravenous sonographic contrast agent: experimental studies. J Ultrasound Med 1993; 12:463–70.

14. Fobbe F, Ohnesorge O, Reichel M, Ernst O, Schuermann R, Wolf K. Transpulmonary contrast agent and color-coded duplex sonography: first clinical experience. Radiology 1992; 185(P):142.

15. Unger E, Shen D, Fritz T, et al. Gas-filled lipid bilayers as ultrasound contrast agents. Invest Radiol 1994; 29:134–136.

16. Mattrey RF, Scheible FW, Gosink BB, Leopold GR, Long DM, Higgins CB. Perfluoroctylbromide: a liver/spleenspecific and tumor-imaging ultrasound contrast material. Radiology 1982; 145:759–62.

17. Fritzsch T, Hauff P, Heldmann F, Lüders F, Uhlendorf V, Weitschies W. Preliminary results with a new liver specific ultrasound contrast agent. Ultrasound Med Biol 1994; 20:137.

18. Mattrey RF, Leopold GR, van Sonnenberg E, Gosink BB, Scheible FW, Long DM. Perfluorochemicals as liver- and spleenseeking ultrasound contrast agents. J Ultrasound Med 1983; 2:173–6.

19. Chin CT, Burns PN. Predicting the Acoustic Response of a Microbubble Population for Contrast Imaging. Ultrasound Med Biol 2000; In press.

20. de Jong N. Physics of Microbubble Scattering. In: Nanda NC, Schlief R, Goldberg BB, eds. Advances in Echo Imaging Using Contrast Enhancement. Dubai: Kluwer Academic Publishers, 1997:39–64.

21. Apfel RE, Holland CK. Gauging the Likelihood of Cavitation From Short-Pulse, Low-Duty Cycle Diagnostic Ultrasound. Ultrasound Med Biol 1991; 17:175–185.

22. von Bibra H, Sutherland G, Becher H, Neudert J, Nihoyannopoulos P. Clinical evaluation of left heart Doppler contrast enhancement by a saccharide-based transpulmonary contrast agent. The Levovist Cardiac Working Group. J Am CollCardiol 1995; 25:500–8.

23. Uhlendorf V. Physics of ultrasound contrast imaging: scattering in the linear range. IEEE Trans UFFC 1994; 41:70–79.

24. Burns PN, Powers JE, Hope Simpson D, et al. Harmonic power mode Doppler using microbubble contrast agents: an improved method for small vessel flow imaging. Proc IEEE UFFC 1994:1547–1550.

25. Bleeker H, Shung K, Barnhart J. On the application of ultrasonic contrast agents for blood flowmetry and assessment of cardiac perfusion. J Ultrasound Med 1990; 9:461–71.

26. Neppiras EA, Nyborg WL, Miller PL. Nonlinear behaviour and stability of trapped micron-sized cylindrical gas bubbles in an ultrasound field. Ultrasonics 1983; 21:109–115.

27. Burns PN, Powers JE, Fritzsch T. Harmonic imaging: a new imaging and Doppler method for contrast enhanced ultrasound. Radiology 1992; 185(P):142 Abstr).

28. Burns PN, Powers JE, Hope Simpson D, Uhlendorf V, Fritzsch T. Harmonic contrast enhanced Doppler as a method for the elimination of clutter – In vivo duplex and color studies. Radiology 1993; 189:285.

29. Mulvagh SL, Foley DA, Aeschbacher BC, Klarich KK, Seward JB. Second harmonic imaging of an intravenously administered echocardiographic contrast agent: Visualization of coronary arteries and measurement of coronary blood flow. J Am Coll Cardiol 1996; 27:1519–25.

30. Porter TR, Xie F, Kricsfeld D, Armbruster RW. Improved myocardial contrast with second harmonic transient ultrasound response imaging in humans using intravenous perfluorocarbon-exposed sonicated dextrose albumin. J Am Coll Cardiol 1996; 27:1497–501.

31. Kono Y, Moriyasu F, Yamada K, Nada T, Matsumura T. Conventional and harmonic grey-scale enhancement of the liver with sonication activation of a US contrast agent. Radiology 1996; 201.

32. Burns PN, Wilson SR, Muradali D, Powers JE, Fritzsch T. Intermittent US harmonic contrast enhanced imaging and Doppler improves sensitivity and longevity of small vessel detection. Radiology 1996; 201:159.

33. Becher H. Second harmonic imaging with Levovist: initial clinical experience, Second European Symposium on Ultrasound Contrast Imaging. Rotterdam, 1997. Erasmus Univ.

34. Kaul S. Myocardial contrast echocardiography in coronary artery disease: potential applications using venous injections of contrast. Am J Cardiol 1995; 75:61–68.

35. Hamilton MF, Blackstock DT. Nonlinear Acoustics. San Diego: Academic Press, 1998.

36. Burns PN, Hope Simpson D, Averkiou MA. Nonlinear Imaging. Ultrasound Med Biol 2000; In press.

37. Burns PN, Wilson SR, Muradali D, Powers JE, Greener Y. Microbubble destruction is the origin of harmonic signals from FS069. Radiology 1996; 201:158.

38. Hope Simpson D, Chin CT, Burns PN. Pulse Inversion Doppler: A new method for detecting nonlinear echoes from microbubble

contrast agents. IEEE Transactions UFFC 1999; 46:372–382.

39. Tiemann K, Lohmeier S, Kuntz S, et al. Real-time contrast echo assessment of myocardial perfusion at low emission power: first experimental and clinical results using power pulse inversion imaging. Echocardiography 1999; 16:799–809.

40. Porter TR, Xie F. Transient myocardial contrast after initial exposure to diagnostic ultrasound pressures with minute doses of intravenously injected microbubbles. Demonstration and potential mechanisms. Circulation 1995; 92:2391–5.

41. Uhlendorf V, Scholle F-D. Imaging of spatial distribution and flow of microbubbles using nonlinear acoustic properties. Acoustical Imaging 1996; 22:233–238.

42. Taylor KJ, Burns PN, Wells PNT. Clinical Applications of Doppler Ultrasound. New York: Raven Press, 1996.

43. Brennan CE. Cavitation and Bubble Dynamics. New York: Oxford University Press, 1995.

44. Poritsky H. The collapse or growth of a spherical bubble or cavity in a viscous fluid, First U.S. National Congress on Appl. Mech, 1951.

45. Rayleigh L. On the Pressure Developed in a Liquid During the Collapse of a Spherical Cavity. Philosophy Magazine 1917; Series 6:94–98.

46. Plesset MS. The dynamics of cavitation bubbles. J. Appl. Mech. 1949; 16:272–282.

47. Child SZ, Hartman CL, Schery LA, Carstensen EL. Lung Damage from Exposure to Pulsed Ultrasound. Ultrasound in Medicine and Biology 1990; 16:817–825.

48. Miller MW, Miller DL, Brayman A. A Review of in Vitro Bioeffects of Inertial Ultrasonic Cavitation From a Mechanistic Perspective. Ultrasound Med Biol 1996; 22:1131–1154.

49. Miller DL, Gies RA, Chrisler WB. Ultrasonically Induced Hemolysis at High Cell and Gas Body Concentrations in a Thin-Disk Exposure Chamber. Ultrasound Med Biol 1997; 23:625–633.

50. Miller DL, Thomas RM, Williams AR. Mechanisms for Hemolysis By Ultrasonic Cavitation in the Rotating Exposure System. Ultrasound Med Biol 1991; 17:171–178.

51. Miller DL, Thomas RM. Ultrasound Contrast Agents Nucleate Inertial Cavitation in Vitro. Ultrasound Med Biol 1995; 21:1059–1065.

52. Holland CK, Roy RA, Apfel RE, Crum LA. In Vitro Detection of Cavitation Induced by a Diagnostic Ultrasound System. IEEE Trans. IEEE Transaction on Ultrasonics, Ferroelectrics, and Frequency Control 1992; 29:95–101.

53. Everbach EC, Makin IRS, Francis CW, Meltzer RS. Effect of Acoustic Cavitation on Platelets in the Presence of an Echo-Contrast Agent. Ultrasound Med Biol 1998; 24:129–136.

54. Williams AR, Kubowicz G, Cramer E. The Effects of the Microbubble Suspension SHU 454 (Echovist) on Ultrasound-Induced Cell Lysis in a Rotating Tube Exposure System. Echocardiography 1991; 8:423–433.

55. Uhlendorf V, Hoffmann C. Nonlinear acoustical response of coated microbubbles in diagnostic ultrasound. Proc IEEE Ultrasonics Symp 1994:1559–1562.

56. Lanza GM, Wallace KD, Scott MJ, et al. Initial description and validation of a novel site targeted ultrasonic contrast agent. Circulation 1995; 92:I–260.

57. Christy DH, Wallace KD, Lanza GM, et al. Quantitative intravascular ultrasound: demonstration using a novel site targeted acoustic contrast agent. Proc IEEE Ultrasonics Symp 1995:1125–1128.

58. Unger EC. Drug delivery applications of ultrasound contrast agents, Second European Symposium on Ultrasound Contrast Imaging. Rotterdam, 1997. Erasmus Univ.

59. Greenleaf WJ, Bolander ME, Sarkar G, Goldring MB, Greenleaf JF. Artificial Cavitation Nuclei Significantly Enhance Acoustically Induced Cell Transfection. Ultrasound Med Biol 1998; 24:587–595.

60. Unger EC, McCreery TP, Sweitzer RH. Ultrasound Enhances Gene Expression of Liposomal Transfection. Investigative Radiology 1997; 32:723–727.

2 Assessment of Left Ventricular Function by Contrast Echo

And they shall be accounted poet kings
Who simply tell the most heart-easing things

John Keats 1795–1821

2.1 Physiology and pathophysiology of LV function

Accurate and reproducible quantification of left ventricular (LV) function is a crucial component of clinical cardiology. LV function should be assessed in each cardiac patient. Earlier, research and development of diagnostic measures concentrated on systolic LV function, because diastole was thought to be a passive process, which is now known not to be the case. However, it is still easier to evaluate systolic than diastolic function. In the physiology lab, LV function is assessed using calculations derived from pressure and volume recordings; in clinical cardiology measurement of LV wall motion has become the usual method for routine invasive and non-invasive diagnostics (1). We distinguish between global and regional systolic function; in order to assess global systolic LV function, quantification of end-diastolic and end-systolic volumes (LVED, LVES) and ejection fraction (EF) is essential. LV volume and ejection fraction are powerful prognostic measures in patients with coronary and valvular heart disease (2).

Regional LV function is assessed by imaging individual segments of the left ventricle. Wall thickening and the extent of active wall motion are evaluated. Regional function is crucial in the diagnosis of ischemic heart disease. Since reduced perfusion results in wall motion abnormality, impaired regional function can be used as an indicator of perfusion deficits. However, there is a perfusion threshold above which wall motion abnormalities become apparent. Animal experiments have shown that wall motion is normal if less than 20 percent of the thickness of the myocardium is involved or if the circumferential extent of the ischemia (infarction) is less than 12 percent of the entire circumference. Transmural infarctions involving less than 5 percent of the left ventricular mass may be below the threshold to produce detectable wall abnormality (3).

Diastolic LV function is determined by the filling of the left ventricle by means of a complex process involving passive and active components. Since reliable measurement of wall motion in diastole is more difficult than in systole, information on intracardiac pressures is needed. For non-invasive studies, Doppler velocities at the mitral valve and in the pulmonary vein (PV) are correlated to direct hemodynamic pressure recordings (4) (Figure 1). Diastolic dysfunction is increasingly recognised as a key cause of heart failure symptoms in many patients whose systolic function is normal. Abnormalities in diastolic function occur within seconds of the onset of coronary occlusion. Shortly afterwards, wall thickening and endocardial motion are impaired (5). In chronic ischemia or myocardial disease, diastolic dysfunction may be found without systolic dysfunction; patients are not correctly treated if only systolic dysfunction is evaluated.

Assessment of systolic LV function by echocardiography	
Regional LV function	Global LV function
Wall thickening/ endocardial movement	End-diastolic/end-systolic volumes, ejection fraction
Apical and parasternal views: ASE standard, 6 segments/scanplanes	2 or 3 apical scanplanes
Usually qualitative	Mostly quantitative

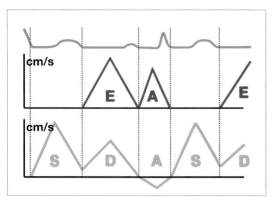

Fig. 1 Schema of normal relation of mitral flow (top) and pulmonary venous flow (bottom). E = early diastolic LV filling, A = filling following atrial contraction, S = systolic antegrade flow, D = diastolic antegrade flow, A = retrograde flow during atrial contraction.

2.2 Available methods – The role of contrast

2.2.1 Systolic function: the need for endocardial border definition

Two-dimensional echocardiography is the method of choice for evaluating systolic LV function. Visual assessment of wall thickening and inward motion of the endocardium is mostly used to assess regional and global LV function. The dynamics of regional wall motion are usually assessed visually using semiquantitative grading *(dyskinetic, akinetic, hypokinetic or normal)*. Similarly global LV function is assessed visually *(normal, low, medium or severe)*. LV volumes and ejection fraction are not measured in routine clinical practice due to difficulties in obtaining reliable data. The prerequisite for reliable measurements is visibility of the entire endocardium in cross section, which can present a problem, particularly on still frames. Dropouts and noise in the image may impair endocardial definition. For the same reasons, the application of automatic quantification and three-dimensional (3 D) reconstruction is still limited. Endocardial borders can be assessed more satisfactorily with moving images, therefore many institutions use a semiquantitative visual scale rather than manually tracing the endocardium and calculating the numerical volumes (6). Nonetheless, accurate and reproducible quantification of left ventricular ejection fraction should be the aim of every study which evaluates LV function.

Transesophageal echocardiography (TEE) provides excellent endocardial definition in most patients, but off-axis imaging may present difficulty (7). Because reliable less invasive and alternatives are available, the indication for a TEE is rarely a simple assessment of LV function, except in mechanically ventilated patients in the intensive care unit. Moreover, stress studies are impractical and inconvenient using the transesophageal approach.

Methods for measurement of systolic LV function

- Fundamental/harmonic B-mode imaging
- Transesophageal echocardiography (TEE)
- Pulsed wave Doppler echocardiography
- Contrast echocardiography
- Nuclear gated blood-pool imaging
- Magnetic resonance imaging (MRI)
- Cine left ventriculography

Non-echocardiographic methods suffer from the same limitations of sensitivity in detecting wall motion abnormalities (8–10). The advantage of scintigraphy (and of MRI and angiography) is that the acquisition of the images is much less observer-dependent than in echocardiography. Moreover, non-echocardiographic methods work in patients for whom ultrasound methods fail because of a poor acoustic window. Scintigraphy and angiography have been validated in numerous trials. Nuclear gated blood-pool imaging is considered the gold standard for assessment of LV function because it provides a 3 D data set for quantification of LV volumes and ejection fraction. Nevertheless, gated blood pool scintigraphy is relatively costly for the data obtained and it is now used more as a reference method to validate new echocardiographic methods (11). In clinical practice there is no real alternative to echocardiography, which is widely available, portable and repeatable. The introduction of contrast media has further reduced the need for non-echocardiographic methods. Opacification of the left ventricle has been shown to enhance endocardial border definition in a series of well documented studies (12–16). A significant number of suboptimal exams have been salvaged using intravenous contrast injections. In combination with stress echocardiography, contrast agents greatly enhance quantification of LV function. It is more difficult to obtain satisfactory images during stress even in patients with good acoustic windows. In several studies both inter- and intra-observer variability decreased significantly with the addition of contrast agents.

With conventional imaging methods, as many as 20 percent of echocardiographic studies may be suboptimal for reliable subjective assessment of left ventricular function. With the advent of tissue harmonic imaging, this figure has fallen to 5–10 percent (17). Ongoing improvement of ultrasound systems will result in further improvement of image quality, so there will be less need in future for contrast to improve visual assessment of LV wall motion.

However, automatic border delineation works much better with contrast enhanced images, especially in colour or power Doppler modes.

2.2.2 Diastolic function: the need for pulmonary venous flow recordings

Diastolic function is still neglected in many routine studies. If measured at all, flow at the mitral valve level is recorded and the ratio of E to A wave amplitudes is used. It is well known that this approach is simplistic and pulmonary venous flow data are needed to avoid misinterpretation of findings derived exclusively from pulsed wave Doppler tracings of the mitral flow (18). In addition to diastolic LV function, the combined use of mitral and pulmonary venous flow curves has proved useful for distinguishing between restrictive and constrictive LV dysfunction, allowing analysis of the severity of mitral regurgitation and detection of atrial parasystole after heart transplantation.

The problem with transthoracic recordings of pulmonary venous flow is that these tracings cannot satisfactorily be obtained in many adult patients. Weak and noisy signals are often found in patients with poor acoustic windows due to obesity or emphysema. TEE is an alternative to a certain extent, but it is semi-invasive, time-consuming and is usually not performed only to assess diastolic function. Contrast enhancement to rescue weak Doppler signals is now the method of choice for obtaining satisfactory PV flow recordings in patients who are difficult to image (19, 20). In the future, tissue Doppler may be an alternative, but at least for the moment, moderately good acoustic windows are needed for reliable tissue Doppler studies. The strength of this method lies in the segmental analysis of LV diastolic function. Recent studies give reference values for this new method, but its clinical importance compared to traditional Doppler methods has yet to be established.

2.3 Indications and selection of methods

2.3.1 Indications for contrast echo

Endocardial border visualisation score	
0	Not visible
1	Barely visible
2	Well visualised

2.3.1.1 LV border delineation

A simple three step visual score can be used to grade the quality of endocardial border definition (Figure 2). Using the 22 segment model of the American Society of Echocardiography (ASE), a suboptimal B-mode echocardiogram is defined as a study in which more than two segments are classified as 1 or 0. Contrast echocardiography should always be performed if the recordings obtained with the usual basic techniques or tissue harmonic imaging – if available – are suboptimal (Figure 3). There is sufficient evidence that endocardial delineation is improved using an ultrasound contrast agent both for fundamental echocardiography and harmonic imaging (11–16, 21, 22). However, the use of contrast should only be contemplated if the anticipated improvement in endocardial delineation changes the way in which the patient is further treated. Not every patient with incomplete endocardial delineation deserves a contrast examination. In the case of an 80-year old patient, for example, apical hypokinesia by itself is often indicative even when the lateral wall is poorly displayed.

In clinical practice, there are two groups of patients for whom contrast echocardiography is of immediate diagnostic benefit: the first are patients on intensive care wards where a reliable assessment of LV function is vital. These patients are often difficult to image because of their limited mobility or mechanical ventilation. Transesophageal echocardiography is often necessary in such situations. Contrast echocardiography is a cheap and time-saving alternative to the considerably lengthier and more invasive TEE examination, particularly as there is always access to a vein in these patients and contrast echocardiography prolongs the usual transthoracic ultrasound examination by only a few minutes.

Stress echocardiography is another ultrasound examination in which the administration of contrast does not prolong the examination unduly but in which there may be a useful gain in diagnostic confidence. In the case of

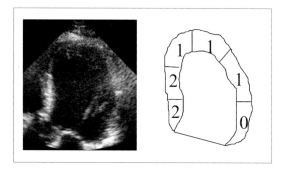

Fig. 2 Four chamber view showing different degrees of endocordial border delineation for the single myocardial segments, judgment using a three step LV endocardial delineation score.

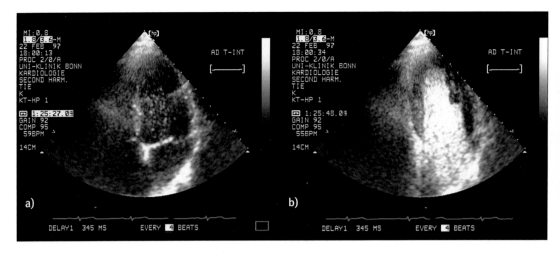

Fig. 3 Suboptimal non-contrast four chamber view (a), with poorly visualised endocardial border of the lateral wall. Following 4 ml Levovist (400 mg/ml), the left ventricle is fully opacified and endocardial borders are clearly defined.

pharmacological stress, access to a vein is made through which the contrast agent can be administered. It is a waste of time to try to analyze changes in wall motion – which are often marginal – with special equipment and time consuming protocols in patients with suboptimal images! Only when endocardial borders are well delineated can reproducible and useful results be expected with this method (6). If a patient does not have a good acoustic window, stress echocardiography should not be performed today without contrast enhancement. The total costs of a stress echo with contrast agent are well below those of a myocardial scintigram which is used to diagnose ischemia and vitality when patients are difficult to image.

2.3.1.2 Detection, determination of size and shape of LV thrombi

Recent observations, though few in number, have demonstrated convincingly the usefulness of LV opacification for delineation of thrombi (23, 24). It is difficult to offer general recommendations for a technique based on these studies. Our own experience, however, suggests that contrast enhanced pulse inversion imaging or harmonic power Doppler will often enhance the visibility of LV thrombi if fundamental or tissue harmonic B-mode are equivocal (Figure 4).

Contrast for LV opacification

When to use contrast

- Assessment of LV function in patients with suboptimal recordings in 2–6 segments
- Automatic LV boundary detection and 3 D reconstruction
- Delineation of LV thrombi

When *not* to use contrast

- If anticipated image improvement will not alter patient management
- If native recordings are adequate
- If native recordings are irredeemably inadequate

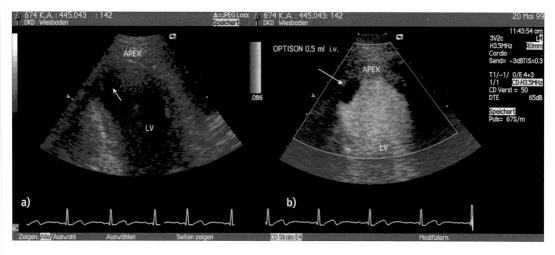

Fig. 4 Apical four chamber view, noise in the apex using harmonic B-mode without contrast (left), delineation of a thrombus impossible; the right panel shows a nice delineation of an apical thrombus using triggered harmonic power Doppler and injection of 0.5 ml Optison.
Courtesy of Heinz Lambertz, Deutsche Klinik für Diagnostik Wiesbaden, Germany

2.3.1.3 Pulmonary venous flow

Administration of contrast to enhance pulmonary venous Doppler should be considered for all patients presenting with heart failure and normal systolic LV function, for whom native Doppler curves are non-diagnostic. Suspected tamponade and restrictive or constrictive cardiac disease are rare but important indications (18). Systolic function may be normal under these conditions and other Doppler parameters not indicative. In this case we recommend contrast enhanced Doppler for every patient who gets contrast for LV opacification or myocardial perfusion. The study can be performed during washout and improves recordings and diagnostic confidence even in those patients who already have diagnostic baseline recordings.

When to use contrast to enhance pulmonary venous Doppler

In patients with suboptimal PV Doppler waveforms

- Patients with heart failure but normal systolic function
- Patients with suspected restrictive or constrictive disease
- Patients with suspected tamponade

In patients who receive contrast for LVO or myocardial perfusion

- All patients. PV signals obtained during wash-out of contrast are improved in all cases

---

2.3.2 Selection of patients

Contrast cannot rescue LV delineation studies when native images are totally inadequate. The maximum yield of contrast enhancement has been demonstrated in patients in whom endocardial borders of 2–6 segments are not delineated satisfactorily. However, with a excellent delineation of endocardial borders, they are limited by a reduced frame rate compared to B-mode harmonics and by wall motion artifacts. For these reasons harmonic B-mode is first choice for assessment of LV wall motion. If continuous colour Doppler is still not able to opacify LV cavity completely, using this method in triggered mode usually provides complete LV opacification and at least provides information on ejection fraction. In the rare event that all transthoracic ultrasound methods fail, TEE or scintigraphy should be used.

2.4 How to perform an LV contrast study

2.4.1 Fundamental B-mode

Fundamental (conventional) imaging should only be used when harmonic imaging is not available. While perfluorocarbon agents such as Optison, Definity or SonoVue provide adequate signal to produce opacification in fundamental mode, Levovist does not (Figure

Fundamental B-mode for LVO: settings

Initial settings for all systems (preset):

Scanhead frequency	2.5 – 3.5 MHz
Transmit power	Mechanical index (MI) < 0.6
Dynamic range	Low – medium
Line density	Medium or high
Compression	Medium – high
Persistence	Disabled

Individual adjustment of instrument controls:

Transmit power	Try reduction of initial level if apical swirling (due to bubble destruction) is seen
Scanplanes	Conventional planes
Focus	Below mitral valve (apical planes), below posterior wall (parasternal view), to reduce bubble destruction in the near field
Time gain compensation	As in fundamental imaging
Lateral gain (HP only)	As in fundamental imaging
Receive gain	Slightly reduce gain to decrease the grey levels in the myocardium before injection of contrast

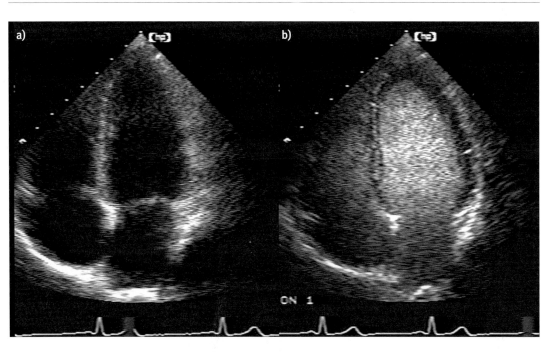

Fig. 7 Apical four chamber view using fundamental B-mode before and after injection of 10 μl/kg of Definity. Poor endocardial endocardial definition without contrast (a), good opacification and delineation of the cavity following contrast injection (b).
Courtesy of Neil J Weissman, Washington Hospital Center, Washington DC, USA

7). Harmonic imaging allows lower dose, with consequently less attenuation artifact and longer duration (Figure 8). Conversion of non-diagnostic to diagnostic echocardiograms with contrast is possible in many patients, but still about 30 percent of suboptimal studies cannot be salvaged with fundamental contrast echo. The contrast dose for fundamental imaging is about 3 times higher than for harmonic imaging. As with harmonic imaging, adjustment of transmit power is crucial for optimal contrast effect. When switching from non-contrast imaging to a contrast study, transmit power should be reduced to limit bubble disruption. The receive gain should be reduced slightly to lower the grey levels in the myocardium before injection of contrast. This enhances the delineation of the cavities. For opacification of the left ventricle, the presence of contrast is more important than differences between contrast signal amplitudes. Therefore dynamic range can be set low and the compression raised slightly.

2.4.1.1 Contrast agent dose

Optison: 1.0 ml as a bolus, followed by a rapid flush of saline (5 ml). The injection rate should not exceed 1 ml per second. This dose regimen usually allows sampling of at least 5 cardiac cycles in several imaging planes. If the contrast enhancement is inadequate after the initial dose, a second dose of 2 ml may be injected intravenously. The maximum total dose should not exceed 8.7 ml.

Definity: 10 μl/kg as a bolus. During stress echocardiography, additional injections are

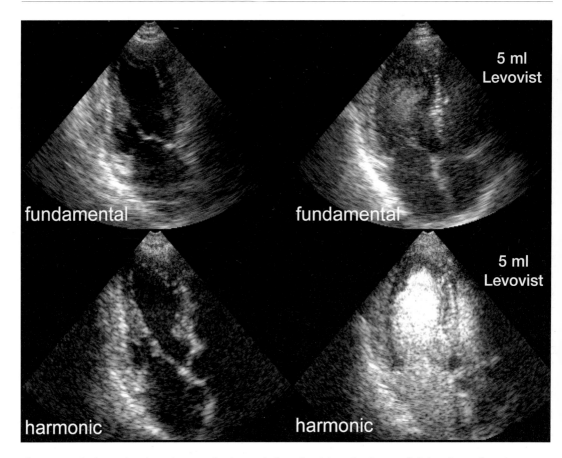

Fig. 8 Apical two chamber view acquired at end-diastole with native frames (left hand panel) and contrast enhanced frames (right hand panel) following intravenous injection of 5 ml Levovist (400 mg/ml). The top images are acquired during fundamental imaging, the bottom images during harmonic imaging. Note the marked improvement of contrast strength of harmonic imaging compared to fundamental imaging.

necessary at peak stress or when the patient becomes symptomatic. Use the same dose as at baseline.

2.4.1.2 Image acquisition and interpretation

Start scanning from an apical window to record the four chamber view. With bolus injections attenuation is usually observed initially. When attenuation subsides and the entire cavity is opacified, check for apical bubble disruption and make a final adjustment to the transmit power. After optimisation, sample at least 5 cardiac cycles (storing to cineloop and/or MO disk) and then record at least another apical view. Parasternal views should always be recorded later, because attenuation by the RV often impairs LV opacification. Evaluation of the stored images is performed as with non-contrast echocardiography.

2.4.1.3 Pitfalls and troubleshooting

The problems and their management are the same as for harmonic B-mode (see §2.4.3).

2.4.2 Fundamental pulsed wave (PW) Doppler

Venous injection of contrast leads to better pulmonary venous flow signals recorded by transthoracic Doppler (Figure 9, 10). A European multicentre study with Levovist has shown that non-diagnostic noisy recordings could be improved by contrast enhancement to enable quantitative assessment (19). There are considerably more transthoracic studies which clearly display the retrograde flow during atrial systole with contrast than without. The peak antegrade and retrograde velocities obtained by transthoracic contrast enhanced Doppler are comparable to those of the TEE technique without an echo-enhancing agent. The dose needed for enhancement of Doppler signals is low compared to that used for LV opacification or perfusion imaging.

Doppler studies for assessment of diastolic LV function include recordings of transmitral flow and pulmonary venous flow. Usually the PW Doppler study at the mitral valve provides adequate signals without contrast enhancement even in patients with poor windows. Contrast enhancement may cause spectral blooming and lead to an unreliable spectral envelope. Therefore the mitral flow signals should be obtained immediately before or late after application of echo contrast. Contrast enhancement will improve both colour Doppler and spectral Doppler signals of pulmonary venous flow. Colour Doppler imaging helps to find the pulmonary veins and align the beam to the vein, but quantitative information is obtained from the pulsed Doppler spectra.

Contrast enhanced studies can be carried out with all commercially available scanners with PW capability. Harmonic imaging is not usually necessary, because tissue motion is rarely a problem. Low frequency transducers (2.5 MHz or less) are preferable because of their sensitivity to flow, but 3.5 MHz transducers have been shown to be effective too. Enhancement of Doppler signals is the contrast method which requires the fewest instrument adjustments. Only the receive gain needs to be adjusted; a

Fundamental pulsed Doppler for pulmonary venous flow enhancement: settings

Initial settings for all systems (preset):

Scanhead	Lowest frequency
Transmit power	Lowest setting consistent with good signals
Scanplanes	Normal
PRF	Normal setting
Sample volume	Normal setting
Scanplanes	Normal setting, no change necessary for contrast
Receive gain	Usually reduction necessary

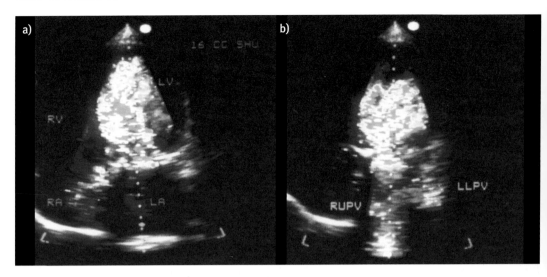

Fig. 9 Contrast enhanced colour Doppler recordings of pulmonary venous flow (four chamber view): no colour Doppler signals in the pulmonary veins without contrast (a), following bolus injection of 5 ml Levovist (300 mg/ml) flow signals in two pulmonary veins, LLPV = left lower pulmonary vein, RUPV = right upper pulmonary vein (b).

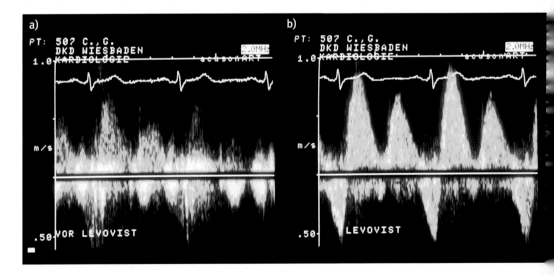

Fig. 10 PW-Doppler-recordings before and after contrast enhancement with 2 ml Levovist (300 mg/ml): in the pre-contrast recording (a) the Doppler spectrum is noisy and not completely displayed, whereas the contrast enhanced recording (b) provides the complete envelope of the Doppler spectrum with high signal to noise ratio. *Courtesy of Heinz Lambertz, Deutsche Klinik für Diagnostik Wiesbaden, Germany*

reduction is usually necessary to avoid spectral blooming and saturation.

According to the *Canadian Consensus Recommendations for the Measurement and Reporting of Diastolic Dysfunction*, the right upper pulmonary vein is evaluated using the four chamber view (18). After parallel alignment of the beam to the vein in colour Doppler mode PW Doppler interrogation is initiated adjusting the gain in the same way as without contrast. The receive gain should be adjusted in most patients because the optimal dose for the individual patient cannot be predicted. The recommended dose of echo contrast is sufficient to achieve signal enhancement even in patients with very poor windows. The criteria for an optimal contrast enhanced Doppler spectrum are the same as for non-contrast Doppler studies. Since the sample volume for interrogation of pulmonary venous flow is far from the skin, local acoustic power usually is not high enough to cause significant bubble disruption noise. Therefore no reduction in transmit power is normally needed.

2.4.2.1 Contrast agent dose

If pulmonary venous flow is evaluated together with LV opacification or myocardial perfusion, the wash-out phase can be used for Doppler enhancement and no additional contrast injection is needed.

If enhancement of PV flow is the primary indication, bolus injections of Levovist (3 ml, 300 mg/ml concentration), Optison (0.3 ml) or Definity (5–10 µl/kg) can be injected as a bolus followed by a flush of 5 ml saline. Usually the Doppler gain has to be reduced to keep the grey level of the Doppler spectrum within the normal ranges.

2.4.2.2 Image acquisition and interpretation

This is the same as for non-contrast Doppler studies. When adequate Doppler spectra are visible, recordings are stored in cineloop or on videotape. Peak antegrade and retrograde velocities and velocity-time integrals as well as duration of retrograde flow are measured. Mitral flow curves are recorded before injection of contrast or after the wash-out and evaluated for peak A and E wave velocities, the velocity-time integrals and the duration of the A-wave. The average of at least 3 cardiac cycles is taken.

2.4.2.3 Pitfalls and troubleshooting
Spectral blooming

In a spectral Doppler system, the arrival of the agent has the effect of increasing the grey level intensity of the display. The peak Doppler shift frequency, which corresponds to the maximum flow velocity in the sample volume, remains unaffected. If, however, the power of the Doppler signal tapers steadily to zero at high Doppler shift frequencies, as is commonly the case (25), another form of the blooming artifact occurs. In Figure 11 one can see that the arrival of the contrast agent is accompanied by an apparent increase in the peak systolic frequency. The blood is not, in fact, flowing any faster; it is simply that the enhanced sensitivity of the detection is causing the weaker signals at the higher Doppler shift frequencies to be displayed.

Pitfalls in contrast enhanced PW-Doppler

- Signals too strong: spectral blooming
- Gain too high: spectral blooming
- Signals too weak: inadequate effect
- Contrast dosage too low: inadequate effect
- Contrast dosage too high: attenuation
- Sample volume not properly placed within the vein: no effect

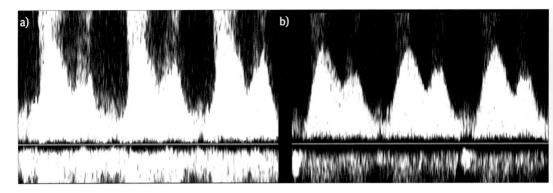

Fig. 11 Spectral blooming of PW Doppler recordings in the right upper pulmonary vein due to inadequate gain setting (a), satisfactory Doppler recording after reduction of gain (b).

Put more concisely, if the dynamic range of the display is not as great as the dynamic range of the signal, the agent will cause the weaker echoes to be displayed preferentially. In most spectral Doppler systems, the same effect can be obtained simply by increasing the Doppler receiver gain setting. Conversely, the artifact can be obviated simply by reducing the Doppler gain setting as the enhancement occurs. The clear conclusion here is that contrast agents should be used to bring undetectable signals into the dynamic range of the display, not to push detectable signals beyond the dynamic range of the display!

Attenuation
Transthoracic imaging of flow in the right upper pulmonary vein is highly dependent on attenuation because of the long distance between transducer and sample volume. This fact often reduces the signal-to-noise ratio in non-contrast Doppler and can be found in contrast enhanced studies if there are too many microbubbles in the left ventricle and atrium. Attenuation is easily identified by switching to harmonic or fundamental B-mode, which will show good opacification in the nearfield but no contrast signals in the deeper parts, particularly in the left atrium. Better penetration of ultrasound can be achieved when the LV contrast appears faint and incomplete. The problem is resolved simply by waiting until further washout has occurred or, if applicable, by reducing the rate of the contrast infusion.

Displaced sample volume
Positioning of the sample volume in contrast enhanced pulsed wave Doppler recordings can be guided by colour Doppler which provides an excellent display of the proximal segment of the right or left upper vein (Figure 9). When the Doppler spectrum is inadequate, the first

Avoiding artifacts in spectral Doppler contrast studies

- Use the agent only if the signal is inadequate because of attenuation by solid tissue. Use the minimum dose needed
- Reduce the Doppler transmitted power to the minimum setting consistent with obtaining a good contrast enhanced signal
- During enhancement, reduce the receive gain to optimise the brightness of the spectral display
- Make velocity measurements only from the optimised display

step should be to check in colour Doppler mode whether the sample volume has been displaced. Underdosing of contrast is rarely the reason when the recommended doses are used. Too low a dosing can be seen in colour Doppler mode (no display of the flow in the pulmonary vein and left atrium) and in B-mode (almost no contrast visible).

2.4.3 Harmonic B-mode

Before a contrast study is considered, non-contrast imaging using tissue harmonic imaging should be tried. In this mode high transmit power is used to enhance tissue signals. For contrast studies, the effect of high transmit power is ambivalent: on the one hand, harmonic response is enhanced and LV contrast signals are more intense; on the other, myocardial grey levels increase, reducing the contrast between LV cavity and myocardial tissue and thus potentially worsening the delineation of endocardial borders. Moreover, bubble disruption is dependent on transmit power and needs to be taken into account when transmit power is adjusted. The following recommendations attempt to balance these opposing effects and have been validated in several studies by different institutions, including ours (16, 21).

2.4.3.1 Contrast agent dose
Levovist: use 4.0 g vials and the 400 mg/ml concentration. Half of the vial is injected as a bolus, followed by a rapid flush of saline.
Optison: 0.5 ml bolus followed by a rapid flush of saline. The injection rate should not exceed 1 ml per second.
These dose regimens usually allow sampling of at least 5 cardiac cycles in several imaging planes. If contrast enhancement is inadequate after the initial dose, a second dose may be injected. The maximum total dose should not exceed 6 vials of Levovist or 8.7 ml Optison. During stress echocardiography additional injections are necessary at peak stress or when the patient becomes symptomatic. Use the same dose as for baseline.

2.4.3.2 Image acquisition and interpretation
Start scanning from an apical window to record the four chamber view. With bolus injections attenuation is usually observed initially. When attenuation subsides and the entire cavity is opacified, check for apical bubble disruption and make a final adjustment to the transmit power. After optimisation, sample at least 5 cardiac cycles (storing to cineloop and/or MO disk) and then record at least another apical view (Figure 12). Parasternal views should always be recorded later, because attenuation by the RV often impairs LV opacification. Evaluation of the stored images is performed as with non-contrast echocardiography.

During dobutamine stress the low amounts of Optison and Definity can be injected into the line without interrupting the infusion of dobutamine. The agent is driven by the dobutamine infusion and provides prolonged LV opacification. For Levovist higher volumes

Pitfalls in contrast harmonic B-mode

- Attenuation
- Blooming
- Bubble dissolution
- Nearfield defects
- Inhomogeneous opacification, swirling
- Systolic reduction/disappearance of contrast
- LVOT defect in aortic regurgitation
- Anti-contrast: myocardium and cavity almost same grey level

Harmonic B-mode for real-time LVO: settings

Initial settings for all systems (preset):

Imaging mode	Pulse inversion (ATL) or harmonic B-mode
Dynamic range	Low – medium
Compression	Medium – high
Line density	Medium
Persistence	Disabled
Transmit power	MI < 0.3 for pulse inversion (ATL)
	MI < 0.6 for all other systems

Individual adjustment of instrument controls:

Transmit power	Reduction if apical defect or swirling is seen, try to increase if global contrast is too weak
Scanplanes	Same as conventional planes
Focus	Below mitral valve (apical planes) or below posterior wall (parasternal view). Reduces bubble destruction in the near field
Receive gain	Slightly reduce gain to decrease the grey levels in the myocardium before injection of contrast
Time gain compensation	As for non-contrast studies
Lateral gain (HP only)	As for non-contrast studies

are necessary, therefore we recommend interruption of the dobutamine infusion and very slow injection (at least 5 seconds) to avoid administration of a dobutamine bolus.

2.4.3.3 Pitfalls and troubleshooting
Bubble disruption
Nearfield defects, inhomogeneous opacification, systolic reduction or disappearance of contrast are all due to bubble disruption. Due to the higher local acoustic pressures close to the transducer, more bubbles are destroyed in the nearfield and during systole where the higher pressures enhance bubble disruption. In apical views swirling may be seen, reflecting mixing of apical blood containing low amounts of microbubbles with blood from deeper regions with more microbubbles (Figure 13). Inadequate contrast effect in the left ventricular outflow tract (LVOT) may be found in

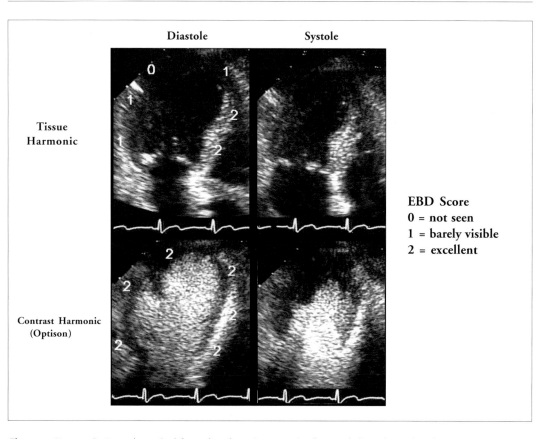

Fig. 12 Harmonic B-mode, apical four chamber view acquired at end-diastole and end-systole with native frames (top images) and contrast enhanced frames (bottom images) following intravenous injection of 0.4 ml Optison.
Courtesy of Sharon Mulvagh, Mayo Clinic, Rochester MN, USA

patients with aortic insufficiency, which also causes increased bubble dissolution. First check to see whether the settings listed in the Table are helpful. The most frequent error is leaving the transmit power on the same level as in tissue harmonic mode and not changing the focus position. Adjusting these parameters often gives satisfactory images. If the instrument controls are correctly set, attempts should be made to reduce the transmit power further. If this measure does not produce better LV opacification, administration of a higher dose of contrast should be considered.

The receive gain is less important. It should be reduced to a level where myocardial tissue only produces weak signals. This can further enhance the differentiation between contrast signals in the cavity and myocardial tissue. However by doing this, the baseline image becomes worse than with a normal non-contrast gain setting. It is important to bear in mind the special distinction between the transmit power and the receive gain controls in a contrast study. The transmit power controls the energy delivered by the scanhead, which determine bubble behaviour, whereas the

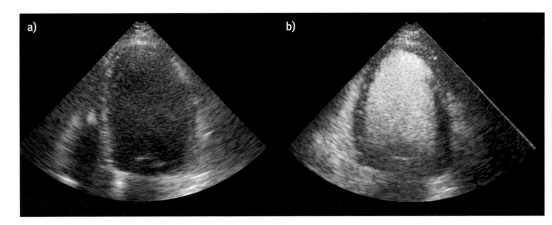

Fig. 13 Apical four chamber view using harmonic B-mode before and after injection of 4 ml Levovist (400 mg/ml). Systolic swirling due to apical bubble destruction (a) can be reduced by decreasing transmit power of the scanhead (lower mechanical index) and increasing receive gain, complete opacification during diastole (b).

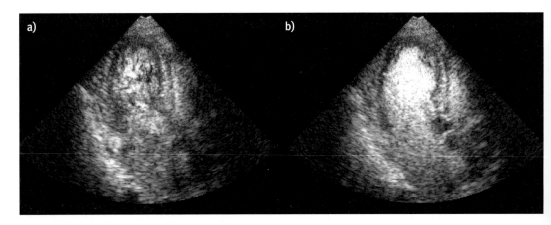

Fig. 14 Apical four chamber view using harmonic B-mode before and after injection of 4 ml Levovist (400 mg/ml). Poor endocardial definition without contrast (a), good opacification and delineation of the cavity following contrast injection. Note that the LV is not completely opacified, particularly below the mitral valve due to contrast shadowing (b).

receive gain simply controls the sensitivity of the scanner to the resulting echo (see §1.3).

Attenuation

Attenuation is often observed following bolus injections of contrast. For a short time there are so many microbubbles in the cavity that the transmitted ultrasound is completely scattered and absorbed by the microbubbles in the near-field and no ultrasound penetrates into the deeper regions of the image. Strong signals are found in the nearfield whereas the deeper parts show no signals (Figure 14). Attenuation subsides with wash-out and waiting for wash-out is the best way to resolve this problem.

> **Impact of transmit power on contrast studies for LV opacification (LVO)**
>
> **Low Power**
> - Low tissue harmonics (myocardium becomes less visible)
> - Low contrast signal intensity
> - Microbubble destruction reduced (homogenous opacification of the entire LV)
>
> **High Power**
> - Strong tissue harmonic (myocardium becomes more visible)
> - High contrast signal intensities
> - Microbubble destruction enhanced (apical filling defects, swirling)

Anti-contrast effect
A specific limitation of all greyscale techniques is the fact that the tissue signals are displayed together with the contrast signals in the LV cavity, from which they cannot sometimes be distinguished. For effective delineation of endocardial borders the amplitudes of the contrast echoes in the cavity should exceed that of the tissue echoes. However, if grey levels within the cavities are comparable to those in the myocardium, an 'anti-contrast' effect is observed (Figure 13 left). The borders of the septum may particularly be obscured because the normal septum is echogenic. In individual still frames, the endocardial border is usually less clear than it is in moving greyscale images. Injection of a higher dose may be considered in order to increase LV contrast in such cases.

2.4.4 Harmonic imaging of LV thrombi

Besides endocardial border delineation contrast echocardiography is useful for delineation of LV thrombi which may be found in conjunction with global or regional wall motion abnormalities. Harmonic imaging without contrast is limited in the nearfield of the transducer because tissue harmonics are weak in the nearfield. High transmit power and nearfield focusing of the beam can be used to enhance display, but sometimes hazy recordings impair reliable confirmation or exclusion of an apical LV thrombus. Real-time pulse inversion using contrast and low transmit power (MI < 0.3) is the method of choice, because it provides the best spatial resolution and apical bubble destruction can be minimised. The other imaging modalities need higher transmit powers with the risk of enhanced apical bubble destruction resulting in false positive findings. With real-time harmonic B-mode, power should be reduced until contrast swirling is absent. Besides apical swirling, the shape of an apical cavity defect reveals whether it is due to apical bubble destruction or an intracavitary mass (Figure 15). Symmetric convex defects suggest bubble destruction rather than thrombi and reduction of the transmit power or higher dose of contrast should be performed.

Harmonic power Doppler works best in destruction mode, which uses high transmit power. Triggered imaging is then necessary to fill the cavity completely. One or two frames per cardiac cycle can be acquired. With all

> **How to avoid artifacts in harmonic B-mode contrast studies**
>
> - Contrast shadowing: wait for wash-out of contrast or lower dose
> - Apical bubble destruction: reduce transmit power
> - Insufficient cavity contrast at all depths: increase dose or use more sensitive imaging method

three imaging modalities the region with a suspected thrombus should be recorded with changing transducer positions, because thrombi are often better displayed with modified scanplanes. Moreover, repeated views have to be obtained during the different phases of LV opacification after injection of the contrast bolus, because high amounts of contrast may obscure thrombi.

> **Imaging LV thrombi with contrast echo**
>
> **Methods**
>
> 1. Real-time pulse inversion using low transmit power (MI < 0.3) (Method of choice: best spatial resolution with minimal apical bubble destruction)
> 2. Real-time harmonic B-mode or triggered harmonic power Doppler (1:1–2)
>
> **Technique**
>
> - Avoid apical destruction of microbubbles by reducing MI
> - Record region with suspected thrombus, changing the transducer position
> - Use modified scanplanes to improve visualisation of thrombus
> - Avoid blooming: record region with suspected thrombus during wash-out of agent

2.4.5 Harmonic colour/power Doppler for LVO

2.4.5.1 Continuous imaging for evaluation of LV wall motion

Although harmonic colour and power Doppler provide the best LV delineation, these techniques are not the first choice for assessment of LV wall motion when non-contrast studies have proved suboptimal. The lower frame rate (typically 10–15 Hz) compared to harmonic B-mode (as high as 50 Hz) and wall motion artifacts limit their use. The frame rate of current colour Doppler systems is simply not sufficient for evaluation of wall motion analysis, particularly during stress with high heart rates. On the other hand, both Doppler techniques are much more sensitive to contrast, so less agent is required if the investigation is performed using Doppler techniques (26–28).

In order to delineate LV cavities, the contrast agent should ideally be visible within the LV cavity but not within the intramyocardial vessels. Using the recommended dose of contrast and machine settings, there should be no significant filling of the intramyocardial vessels (Figure 16, 17). However, the high sensitivity of some newer instruments may cause colour or power Doppler signals within the myocardium. Flow in larger vessels may usually be visible, for instance in the septal perforators, but contrast in smaller subendocardial vessels cannot be displayed with injections of Levovist or Optison using continuous imaging. Thus the endocardial definition is excellent with contrast.

Since continuous colour or power Doppler is usually initiated when harmonic B-mode is suboptimal, the change from one mode to the other should be performed quickly to avoid additional injections of contrast. In most machines you just have to press a button, but optimisation of a few instrument controls is crucial: these settings can be stored as a preset, so they are immediately available (see B-mode settings). If different scanheads are available for harmonic imaging, a lower frequency is usually preferred for Doppler studies because of its greater sensitivity, unlike B-mode, where higher frequencies often work better.

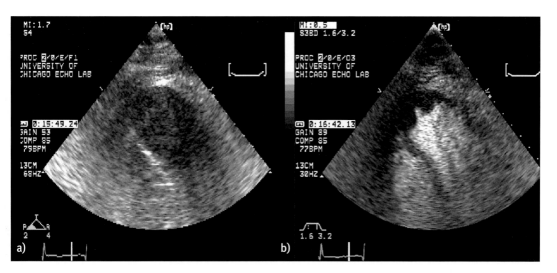

Fig. 15 Harmonic B-mode recordings of a 29-year-old male 2 weeks following an anterior wall myocardial infarction. The study was performed to assess left ventricular performance. Apical four chamber view demonstrates an echo density at the LV apex suspicious for thrombus (a). A multi-lobed apical thrombus is clearly delineated following a bolus injection of Optison (b).
Courtesy of Roberto M Lang, James Bednarz, Victor Mor-Avi and Kirk T Spencer, University of Chicago, Chicago IL, USA

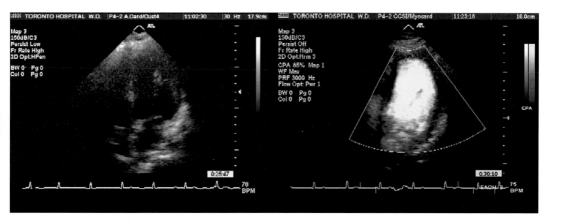

Fig. 16 38-year old patient referred for assessment of left ventricular function prior to the administration of chemotherapy. This patient was unable to complete the assessment of ventricular function by RNA due to claustrophobia and was subsequently referred to the echocardiographic laboratory for the quantitation of left ventricular function. The baseline apical four chamber view is shown using tissue harmonic imaging (THI) (a). Notice that despite the use of THI, endocardial border definition remains poor. After the intravenous injection of 400 mg/ml of Levovist a significant improvement in endocardial border definition is found (b).
Courtesy of Eric Yu, University of Toronto, Canada

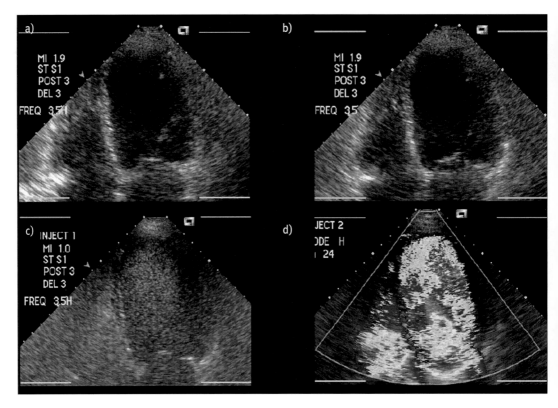

Fig. 17 Endocardial border delineation in a patient with poor acoustic window, comparison of four imaging modes: (a) = fundamental B-mode, (b) = tissue harmonic imaging, (c) = harmonic B-mode and Levovist, (d) = harmonic colour Doppler and Levovist.
Courtesy of of Gian Paolo Bezante, University of Genoa, Italy

Colour Doppler provides information on flow velocity and variance. This information is not needed when colour Doppler is used for LV opacification. The presence of microbubbles in the cavity is of greater interest than their velocity (which will be misestimated if there is bubble destruction anyway). Colour Doppler signals can therefore be displayed in a modified map which uses just one colour. The use of a monochromatic map helps the visual assessment of endocardial borders, particularly in aneurysms.

2.4.5.2 Contrast agent dose

Colour or harmonic power Doppler studies are usually performed during wash-out of contrast injected for harmonic B-mode studies. When Doppler studies are initiated, as soon as LV contrast becomes insufficient for B-mode, no additional contrast has to be injected. Otherwise, additional boluses of contrast may be injected (for instance 5 ml of Levovist at 300 mg/ml concentration).

2.4.5.3 Image acquisition and interpretation

Start scanning with apical windows as for harmonic B-mode. Check for apical bubble destruction and wall motion artifacts. After optimisation, sample at least five cardiac cycles. Then record at least another apical view and

Continuous harmonic colour or power Doppler for LVO: settings

Initial settings for all systems (preset):

Scanhead	Lowest frequency
Transmit power	Mechanical Index (MI) 1.0
	Acuson Sequoia: -6 dB from maximum
Display mode	Colour Doppler
	Standard variance mode (gives a colour mosaic look)
	Unidirectional map (set colour baseline to one flow direction extreme)
	Power Doppler with standard map
Persistence	Disabled
Line density	Highest value
Sensitivity	Medium
Wall filter	Medium
PRF	Highest level

Individual adjustment of instrument controls:

Scanplanes	Same as conventional planes. Optimise in tissue harmonic mode then reduce B-mode receive gain
Power Doppler	Adjust box so that the entire LV-myocardium is included
Focus	Below mitral valve (apical planes), or below posterior wall (parasternal view)
Transmit power	Reduction if apical defect or swirling, try to increase MI if global contrast is too weak
Receive gain	Default, reduce if wall motion artifacts are displayed

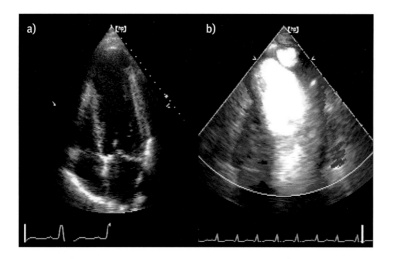

Fig. 18 Two-dimensional image of apparent left ventricular apical aneurysm with suspicious echoes noted at distal lateral wall (a). Harmonic power Doppler contrast image demonstrating flow into a distal lateral pseudoaneurysm (b).
Courtesy of Roberto M Lang, James Bednarz, Victor Mor-Avi and Kirk T Spencer, University of Chicago Chicago IL, USA

parasternal views in the same way. Evaluation of the stored images is performed as for non-contrast echocardiography.

2.4.5.4 Pitfalls and troubleshooting
Same as for triggerd imaging see 2.4.5.8

2.4.6 Triggered imaging for assessment of end-systolic and end-diastolic volumes and ejection fraction

End-diastolic and end-systolic volumes can be measured with continuous imaging by analyzing end-diastolic and end-systolic still frames. If these frames show complete opacification of the LV cavity, reliable measurements can be performed. For those patients with inadequate LV opacification, triggered imaging usually provides opacification of the entire cavity (26, 27).

Triggered or intermittent imaging means that transmission of ultrasound is confined to short time intervals – usually the time to create one single frame. During this period, the microbubbles in the imaging field exhibit their harmonic response and then are rapidly dissolved. Before the next frame is sampled, the microbubbles have to be replenished from areas outside the imaging field. The best way to do this is to interrupt the transmission of ultrasound. Triggered imaging increases the prevalence of microbubbles in the imaging field. The amount of bubbles increases with the duration of the non-transmission periods between the imaging frames. For LV opacifica-

> **Ejection fraction by contrast echo**
>
> High quality, machine-derived LV volume and LVEF measurements can be made in almost all patients using triggered harmonic power or colour Doppler technique.

tion studies only short intervals are necessary and end-systolic and end-diastolic frames can be sampled in the same cardiac cycle.

Bubble destruction presents no problem when triggered imaging is used. Bubbles which are destroyed during imaging produce strong signals which form the basis of the image.

Increasing the transmitted power is actually beneficial to these studies, because it enhances microbubble disruption. At high MI, opacification of the entire LV cavity can be performed even in patients with large aneurysms.

A secondary consequence of a high concentration of microbubbles is the display of intra-

Triggered harmonic colour or power Doppler for LVO: settings

Initial settings for all systems (preset):

Scanhead	Lowest frequency
Transmit power	MI > 1.2
Display mode	Colour Doppler
	Standard variance mode (gives colour mosaic appearance)
	Unidirectional map (set colour baseline to one flow direction extreme)
	Power Doppler with standard map
Persistence	Disabled
Line density	Highest value
Sensitivity	Medium
Wall filter	Medium
PRF	Highest level

Individual adjustment of instrument controls:

Scanplanes	Same as conventional planes. Optimise in tissue harmonic mode then reduce B-mode receive gain
ECG-trigger	End-diastole and end-systole trigger interval every cardiac cycle (use M-mode to set trigger points)
Power Doppler	Adjust box so that entire LV-myocardium is included
Focus	Below mitral valve (apical planes) or below posterior wall (para sternal view)
Transmit Power	MI > 1.2. Do not adjust!
Receive gain	Reduced slightly if myocardial contrast is too high

myocardial contrast. For reliable contour finding of LV volumes, myocardial contrast should be as low as possible. There should be no detectable microbubbles, at least in the smaller subendocardial vessels. Display of larger vessels in the mid or epicardial layers does not, however, interfere with the tracing of the cavity. Because of the short trigger intervals used in the recommended protocol there is unlikely to be visible contrast in the smaller intramyocardial vessels. In addition, the signals derived from smaller intramyocardial vessels are much weaker than the signals found in the cavity. Thus segmentation is possible by limiting the sensitivity of the ultrasound device.

2.4.6.1 Contrast agent dose
Triggered imaging is usually performed in conjunction with continuous harmonic B-mode or harmonic colour/power Doppler, using a bolus injection of contrast. During wash-out there is still enough contrast for triggered colour or power Doppler studies. If assessment of LV ejection fraction is the primary indication, the same dosing scheme is recommended as for assessment of regional wall motion. The benefit of a contrast enhanced segmental wall motion analysis should be exploited in harmonic B-mode, before triggered imaging is initiated.

2.4.6.2 Image acquisition and interpretation
At least two apical views should be recorded. In each view end-systolic and end-diastolic frames of at least five cardiac cycles are recorded and stored on tape or disc. Shallow breathing or breathholding is recommended to acquire comparable planes. Off-line analysis is performed using the software packages implemented in the ultrasound systems. In each view manual tracing of the endocardial borders is performed in at least three cardiac cycles and averaged (Figure 19). Then LVED and LVES volumes are calculated using Simpsons method or the area length method.

2.4.6.3 Pitfalls and troubleshooting
Wall motion artifact
The movement of the myocardial tissue may produce Doppler signals which are different from cavity blooming and from the signals originating from contrast in myocardial vessels (Figure 20). Usually the high pass (wall) filter of the ultrasound system rejects slow-moving structural echoes. However, fast movement of the heart during deep breathing and coughing or exaggerated cardiac motion during physical or dobutamine stress result in wall motion velocities which exceed the threshold of the wall filter. Wall motion artifacts can easily be recognised as flash like coloured areas (changing from frame to frame) which often overlay epi- or pericardial layers of the lateral wall (four chamber view), but may be found in other regions such as near the mitral valve and the septum as well. Structure with high backscatter and fast movement parallel to the beam are prone to produce wall motion artifacts, therefore wall motion artifacts are often found in the fibrotic pericardial layers and the perivalvular tissue.

Note that wall motion artifacts can be seen without contrast! Proper adjustment of the machine settings before contrast injection suppresses most of the signals caused by wall motion. High PRF and wall filter are crucial. Performing the studies with shallow breathing is usually sufficient to prevent wall motion artifacts. If not, patients should hold their breath for 5–10 s. If these measures are not effective, a slightly different scanplane may bring the echodense structures into a position where their movement is more perpendicular to the beam. It is more difficult to suppress wall

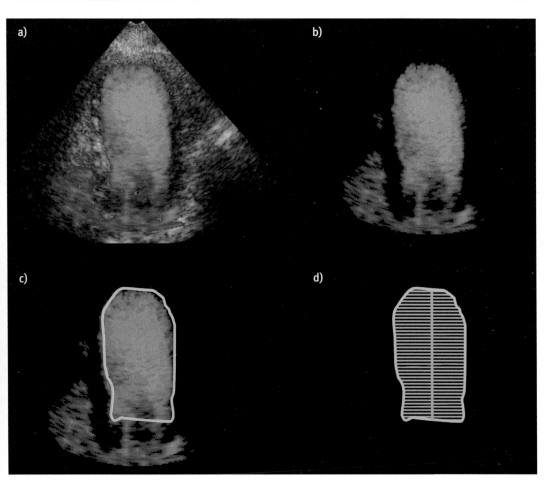

Fig. 19 Tracing of LV borders using harmonic power Doppler imaging. (a) = apical four chamber view acquired at end-diastole, (b) = turning the grey levels to zero, (c) = the contour can easily be traced, (d) = LV cavity contour with Simpsons slices.

motion artifacts during stress. It may be possible to control breathing but the wall motion artifacts caused by increased inotropy may still hinder wall motion analysis.

Myocardial contrast
This is not a real pitfall. With the recommended settings, generally bigger intramyocardial vessels like perforators may be displayed, but these should not be mistaken for wall motion artifacts (see Chapter 3). The reticular or patchy pattern of intramyocardial vessels is very different from more extended wall motion artifacts which often are not confined to myocardial tissue.

Attenuation
When harmonic colour or power Doppler are used during wash-out of a study performed for LV opacification or myocardial perfusion, attenuation will rarely be a problem. In those patients for whom colour Doppler was the

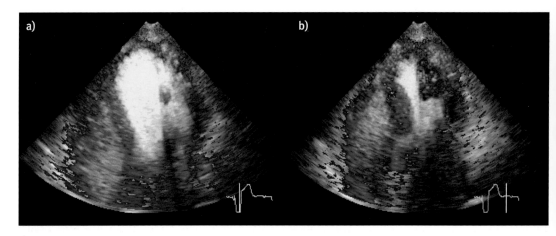

Fig. 20 Myocardial signals during harmonic power Doppler studies for assessment of LV function: end-diastolic (a) and endsystolic (b) frames, endocardial border definition possible despite myocardial signals due to wall motion artifacts (arrows).

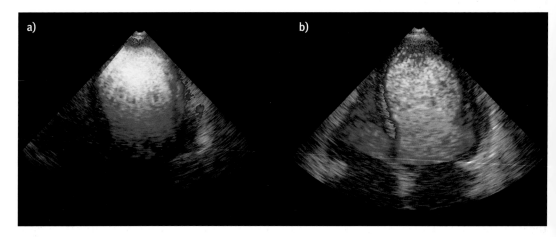

Fig. 21 Harmonic power Doppler: contrast shadowing due to overdosing of contrast (a) with no power Doppler signals at greater depth, better penetration and endocardial border delineation after reduction of infusion rate (b). Note inhomogeneous contrast due to enhanced bubble dissolution in the nearfield.

primary method following injection or infusion of contrast, attenuation may be observed. As with B-mode, strong signals are found in the nearfield whereas the deeper parts show no signals (Figure 21). Attenuation subsides with wash-out and waiting for wash-out is the best way to handle this problem.

Colour blooming

The ultrasound beam used to form an image is not of a precise width, like that of a laser light beam, but tapers in intensity at its edges, more like a flashlight beam. Just as when the intensity of a flashlight beam is increased the illuminated spot it creates appears to get bigger, so when an ultrasound beam encounters a strong scatterer

> **Pitfalls in contrast enhanced harmonic power Doppler**
>
> - Wall motion artifacts
> - Myocardial contrast
> - Attenuation
> - Blooming
> - Bubble disruption

it detects it near the edge of the beam, so interpreting it to be bigger than its actual size. Because of the threshold criterion for colour Doppler images previously described, this effect is especially noticeable in a colour image, where vessels already detected on colour will appear to 'bloom' when the agent arrives. A comparable effect occurs in the axial direction, again because the axial sensitivity of the pulsed Doppler resolution cell is not sharp, but tapers at its proximal and distal boundaries. The effect can be to smother the image with colour, destroying its spatial resolution (Figure 21). In particular, the arrival of contrast in the cavity can cause colour to 'bleed' into the myocardium. It is important that this is not misinterpreted as 'enhanced' detection of flow in the small vessels of the myocardium, nor leads one to overestimate the size of the cavity. Using the minimum dose of the agent that is required to visualise the endocardium is one way to resolve this artifact. Another is to reduce the effective sensitivity of the colour system by either reducing the receiver gain, or, more constructively perhaps, decreasing the ensemble length of the colour detection scheme so that more lines can be made in a shorter time, potentially increasing both the spatial and temporal resolution.

Bubble disruption
Similar to harmonic B-mode, bubble destruction may be a problem in harmonic Doppler modes (which is assessed when apical filling defects are visible or swirling of contrast is observed). The transmit power should then be reduced.

2.5 Summary

Intravenous contrast agents are now approved and available for definition of the left ventricular border and to salvage Doppler recordings in patients who are difficult to image. Extensive studies have demonstrated improvement of image quality and diagnostic confidence, and this is now widely accepted. In spite of this, the the optimal way in which to use contrast deserves consideration . Contrast studies for LV opacification are best performed using contrast specific imaging modalities such as harmonic B-mode, pulse inversion and harmonic power Doppler. Harmonic B-mode provides the highest frame rate which is useful for stress echo, whereas spatial resolution is best using pulse inversion, which enhances delineation of intracardiac masses. Excellent segmentation of the tissue from the cavities on still frames makes harmonic power or colour Doppler the ideal method for measurement of LV volumes and ejection fraction. The protocols and machine

> **Avoiding artifacts in power/colour Doppler contrast studies**
>
> - Use the minimum dose of agent needed
> - Eliminate colour blooming by reducing the Doppler receiver gain
> - Avoid shadowing by imaging after the peak of a bolus or by appropriate titration of the infusion rate
> - If possible, do not image through the right ventricle

3 Assessment of Myocardial Perfusion by Contrast Echocardiography

So much for the circulation! If it is either hindered or perverted or overstimulated, how many dangerous kinds of illnesses and surprising symptoms do not ensue?

William Harvey, De Motu Cordis et Sanguinis, *1578–1657*

Myocardial Perfusion Imaging

No other application of ultrasound contrast agents elicits the enthusiasm evoked by myocardial perfusion imaging. We believe that in the forseeable future contrast echo will replace scintigraphy as the reference method for perfusion imaging. This optimism is based on widespread experience with intracoronary contrast echocardiography where optimal imaging conditions are found. For intravenous contrast perfusion imaging, we hope that the following sections will demonstrate that the technology is ready to yield images of diagnostic quality, but that optimisation and standardisation of clinical approaches are still necessary. This chapter aims to provide a first step.

3.1 Physiology and pathophysiology of myocardial perfusion

3.1.1 Normal perfusion

The vascular compartments in the myocardium comprise the larger arteries, the arterioles, the capillary network and the smaller and larger intramyocardial veins (1) (Figure 1). Following an intracoronary bolus injection of microbubble contrast, an effect is subsequently seen in the different compartments. All currently available echo contrast agents are pure intravascular tracers which traverse the capillary bed of the myocardium following intravenous injection. For assessment of perfusion it is necessary to detect blood in the capillary compartment which contains more than 90 percent of the intramyocardial blood volume.

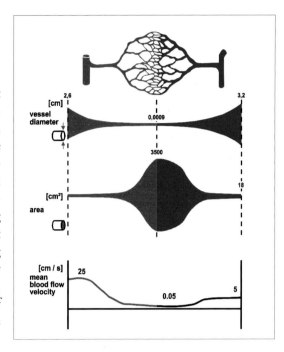

Fig. 1 Scale in the vascular system. 90 percent of the intramyocardial blood volume lies within the capillaries, and this is the objective of the contrast perfusion study. Capillary flow is characterised by velocities of 1 mm/s or less.

Quantitation of perfusion is aimed at measuring the intravascular blood volume and the velocity of blood flow through the vessels, from which flow rate can be derived. Specific techniques are discussed in Chapter 4.

The distribution of intramyocardial vessels is not uniform in the left ventricular (LV) myocardium. Vessel density is highest in the subendocardial layers. Myocardial oxygen consumption of the endocardial layers is higher than that of the epicardial layers, because the endocardium contributes more to wall thickening and is also subject to the highest intramyocardial pressures (2). This spatial non-uniformity of myocardial perfusion is further complicated by the temporal changes in myo-

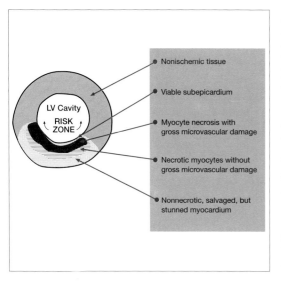

Fig. 2 Acute myocardial infarction showing the subendocardial necrotic zone and viable subepicardial tissue. The extent of wall necrosis increases with length of coronary occlusion and absence of collaterals. *Modified from Braunwald (3).*

myocardial infarction, necrosis occurs first in the subendocardial myocardium (3). With longer occlusions, a front of necrosis moves progressively across the wall involving the transmural thickness of the ischemic zone (Figure 2). The resultant infarct size depends not only on the perfusion bed of the occluded vessel and on the onset of reperfusion, but also on the presence of collateral vessels. After successful recanalisation of an occluded infarct vessel, necrotic zones still have zero flow *(no reflow)*, whereas salvaged myocardium with preserved microvascular integrity is reperfused. It takes some time before mechanical function recovers after an ischemic event. Stunned myocardium is defined as salvaged myocardium which is still akinetic but will regain its contractility within subsequent weeks. The only current diagnostic procedure for early assessment of reperfusion is myocardial scintigraphy.

cardial blood flow (MBF) and myocardial blood volume (MBV). The cyclic changes of MBF are similar to the changes found in the epicardial vessels. The increase in global myocardial blood flow during stress or pharmacological intervention is described in §3.2. Briefly, blood flow through the myocardium can be increased by up to three or four times, provided there is no obstruction in the epicardial or intramyocardial arteries.

3.1.2 Acute myocardial infarction

Transmural myocardial infarction is characterised by areas of significantly reduced or non-existent flow, which has caused necrosis of the myocytes. Myocyte necrosis is associated with necrosis of the vascular cells and local loss of microvascular integrity. During transmural

3.1.3 Chronic ischemic heart disease

At rest, up to 90 percent of stenoses of epicardial vessels do not result in a change in overall MBF in the perfusion bed because of compensatory vasodilation of peripheral vessels. There are, however, differences between the epicardial and subendocardial layers (4). Subendocardial intramural vessels are maximally dilated, whereas subepicardial vessels are not. A vasodilator stimulus will augment transmural flow due to dilation of subepicardial vessels and decrease of the driving pressure. Because subendocardial vessels are already maximally dilated, the fall in driving pressure will result in a fall of flow, whereas subepicardial flow improves and total flow is maintained or increased. Thus the *transmural steal* phenomena from stenosed to normal vessels may be created. However, the transmural gradient is not uniform for a whole hypoperfused segment. Ischemic myocardium can show a heterogeneous pattern with normally perfused areas supplied by collaterals near scars or hypoperfused tissue.

Coronary stenoses may affect the volume of blood within the perfusion bed as well as its blood flow (5). Myocardial blood flow is thought to decrease in the stenosed bed in the presence of hyperemia (6). This decrease may explain the differences in maximal signal intensities between normally and hypoperfused myocardial segments on contrast echo. The reduced blood volume is thought to be brought about by a decrease in capillary density, possibly reflecting the tendency to regulate for a constant capillary perfusion pressure.

3.2 Currently available imaging methods for myocardial perfusion imaging

Perfusion imaging has two major objectives – assessment of ischemia and assessment of myocardial viability. In clinical cardiology there are three established methods to achieve this.

3.2.1 Stress ECG

The probability of a positive stress electrocardiogram (ECG) is only 50 percent in patients with single vessel disease (stenoses > 70 percent) (7, 8). Stress ECG provides only limited information on the extent of ischemia. However, it is the initial method of choice provided there are no contraindications, because it is a simple and inexpensive way of demonstrating inducible myocardial ischemia (Figure 3). If positive, stress ECG can be used for control studies after intervention.

Clinical methods for assessment of myocardial ischemia	
Stress ECG	Limited sensitivity
Stress echocardiography	Wall motion as indirect marker of perfusion
Doppler echocardiography	Limited to LAD perfusion bed
Myocardial scintigraphy	Still the gold standard
Contrast echocardiography	The future ...

3.2.2 Stress echo

Stress echocardiography has become the most important diagnostic method, in spite of the fact that by imaging left ventricular wall motion, it addresses perfusion only indirectly. The sensitivity and specificity are between 80 and 90 percent according to a recent meta-analysis (9). Even under optimal imaging conditions,

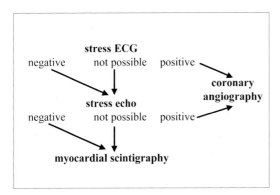

Fig. 3 Traditionally diagnostic path for assessment of inducible ischemia in patients with exertional chest pain and risk factors (University of Bonn).

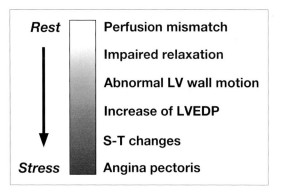

Fig. 4 The ischemic cascade

analysis of LV wall motion is inferior to the display of a perfusion mismatch which precedes the wall abnormality in the ischemic cascade (Figure 4). Classically, flow must be reduced to 50 percent in at least 5 percent of the myocardium to detect new wall motion abnormalities (10). Thus, an echocardiographic perfusion method should enable us to detect myocardial ischemia earlier, providing higher sensitivity in the detection of coronary artery disease. Moreover, there are some important clinical situations in which wall motion cannot be used as an indicator of perfusion. One is the evaluation of patients following thrombolysis of an acute myocardial infarction. Stunned but reperfused myocardium has the same mechanical properties as an unperfused segment, so that clinical decisions cannot be based on wall motion analysis alone.

3.2.3 Coronary flow reserve (CFR)

Doppler echocardiographic measurement of flow at rest and during exercise is a well-validated method for assessment of flow reserve in the left anterior descending (LAD) territory – particularly if contrast enhanced Doppler tracings are used. Coronary flow reserve (CFR) should be included in every perfusion study involving the LAD. However, because of the limitations of the method (§3.12–17) and in order to evaluate the perfusion provided by the circumflex and right coronary arteries, additional methods are needed.

3.2.4 Myocardial scintigraphy

Myocardial scintigraphy is the only established clinical method which directly addresses myocardial perfusion. However, scintigraphy is expensive and is not as widely available as echocardiography. In many European countries scintigraphic studies are not performed in the cardiology department, whereas echocardiographic studies are always carried out in an experienced cardiological setting. Perfusion scintigraphy is known to be less compromised by submaximal stress because perfusion mismatch comes earlier (11, 12). In many centres stress echo is the first choice and scintigraphic studies are confined to patients with poor echocardiographic windows. Theoretically, myocardial scintigraphy should be more sensitive than stress echo in the detection of inducible myocardial ischemia (see Figure 4).

> **Why are wall motion abnormalities not sufficient for the diagnosis of coronary artery disease?**
>
> - Reporting is usually qualitative
> - Perfusion changes preceed wall motion abnormalities
> - Sensitivity and specificity are limited
> - Induction of ischemia is necessary
> - Risk of submaximal stress

In fact, the difference between both methods is marginal due to the technical limitations of scintigraphy (9). Thus the potential of perfusion imaging by contrast ultrasound is not thwarted by scintigraphy. Nevertheless, scintigraphy is widely considered to be the clinical 'gold standard' for perfusion imaging, against which contrast echo will initially be judged. In the future, the roles of the two methods are likely to become complementary.

3.2.5 Myocardial Contrast Echo

There is a clear role for a reproducible, non-invasive, real-time method for imaging myocardial perfusion. Myocardial contrast echo (MCE) offers a pure intravascular tracer, better spatial resolution, the potential for quantitation and real-time imaging during rest, stress and interventional studies. Ultrasound is more widely available, portable and less costly than other methods and remains in the hands of the cardiologist. It is likely to offer complementary diagnostic information to existing methods.

Why myocardial perfusion with echo?

- Better spatial resolution: transmural distribution of perfusion is shown
- Real-time control of imaging
- Uses a pure intravascular tracer
- Inexpensive, portable, uses no ionising radiation
- Patients stay in a specialised cardiological environment.

3.3 Indications and selection of methods

3.3.1 Indications

The potential of contrast echo has been demonstrated in numerous animal studies and humans using intracoronary injections of contrast. However, only few data are available from clinical studies using intravenous injections of contrast. The following guidelines are based on a review of the current literature and on our clinical experience of intravenous contrast echo performed in more than 300 patients over the last three years (13–19). So far there are two clinical situations where we have begun to establish and validate the method:

1. Acute transmural infarction
Contrast echo can be used to determine the infarction size and to assess reperfusion. This indication was the first objective of intracoronary contrast echo, because it can be treated as a yes/no decision (contrast demonstrable versus no contrast) and may be performed without further quantification. Several studies have shown that the area of risk correlates well with that demonstrated using thallium imaging (13). Infarct size and myocardial salvage following reperfusion can be monitored with contrast echocardiography (14). The presence of contrast indicates myocellular viability in patients with recent myocardial infarction (15).

2. Coronary artery stenosis
Detection and functional assessment has been evaluated in preliminary clinical studies (19). Reduction of contrast in a region of interest and reduced velocity of the contrast microbubbles can be used to detect significant

Clinical indications for myocardial contrast echocardiography (MCE) and coronary flow reserve (CFR)

Acute Myocardial Infarction

Prior/post or without coronary angiography:
- Infarct size — MCE
- Reperfusion/no reflow — MCE

Chronic Ischemic Heart Disease

Without coronary angiography:
- Detection of myocardial ischemia (selection for coronary angiography) — MCE

Exclusion of myocardial ischemia*

In conjunction with coronary angiography:
- Functional significance of LAD stenosis — MCE and/or CFR
- Functional significance of other coronary arteries — MCE
- Normal coronary arteries: 'false' positive stress test to confirm cardiac origin of chest pain — CFR
- Microvascular disease — CFR

* Optimal display of the entire myocardium is necessary for this indication, a prerequisite not usually fulfilled with current technology.
** No clinical trials have yet been performed.

---

stenoses of the epicardial vessels during physical and pharmacological stress.

Myocardial contrast echocardiography still suffers from limited display of the myocardium (few scanplanes available, poor imaging conditions in certain regions, see §3.11). It may therefore be questioned whether it is possible to exclude significant stenoses using current technology. However, an abnormal finding in an MCE study, if performed properly, can be taken to represent myocardial ischemia with a reasonable level of confidence. For the time being, MCE should be used in combination with a regular stress echo protocol assessing wall motion abnormalities when detection of inducible myocardial ischemia is the indication. Thus trainees can learn the new method and take advantage of the better sensitivity of MCE compared to wall motion analysis. Should they fail, there still is the data of the established methods. With the introduction of real-time perfusion imaging, wall motion and perfusion can be assessed together, without the present time-consuming combination of imaging modes. This will help facilitate the acceptance of myocardial contrast into the clinical stress echo lab.

Measurement of coronary flow reserve completes an MCE study when the significance of an LAD stenosis has to be evaluated. In patients with normal coronary arteries and chest pain, CFR measurements can be used to confirm or exclude the cardiac origin of the chest pain. Coronary flow reserve provides a quantitative measure whereas reading of MCE studies generally relies on visual assessment. For didactic reasons assessment of CFR is described in a separate section (§3.12). In clinical practice, evaluation of CFR of the LAD should be part of a global perfusion study which includes tissue perfusion. It should be noted that the quantitative approaches for MCE described in Chapter 4 are in rapid development.

cipated from the image quality at baseline. Unlike LV opacification studies, where contrast is indicated for suboptimal baseline imaging, *only* those patients in whom image quality is good should be accepted for a myocardial contrast study. Using tissue harmonic B-mode, patients should have an image quality which would enable a non-contrast stress echo to be successful. For the contrast agent itself, contraindications might rarely result from the specific formulation of the shell or surfactant. For perfusion stress echo, the contraindications are identical to those of a non-contrast study.

3.3.2 Selection of patients and contraindications

With currently available ultrasound equipment and approved contrast agents, we are still working at the margins of the machine's ability to obtain adequate contrast in the myocardial tissue. If the acoustic window is poor, myocardial contrast usually is suboptimal. The success of a contrast study can often be anti-

3.3.3 Selection of the imaging method

Intravenous administration of contrast results in a very low concentration of bubbles in the myocardium which can be evaluated only by using contrast specific imaging modalities. Four contrast specific imaging modes are available (see Table and Chapter 1). All have strengths and weaknesses: some are better suited to per-

Contrast specific imaging methods for assessment of myocardial perfusion				
	Harmonic B-mode	Harmonic power Doppler	Pulse inversion	Power pulse inversion
Bubble-to-tissue sensitivity	Moderate	Very good	Good	Very good
Off-line background subtraction needed	Yes	No	Yes	No
LV-myocardium delineation	Poor	Good	Moderate	Good
Wall motion artifacts	None	Can be severe	Moderate	Few
Real-time imaging	No	No	No	Yes

Perfusion Imaging

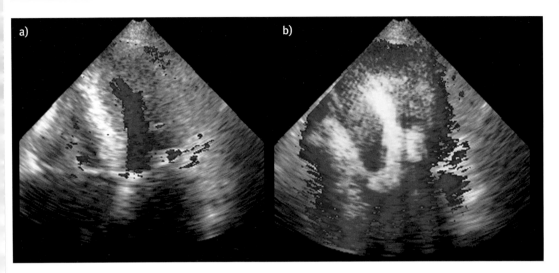

Fig. 5 Harmonic power Doppler recordings (four chamber view) before (a) and during (b) Levovist infusion. Myocardial contrast is clearly visible.

fluorocarbon, some to air-filled microbubbles: some are not available in all scanners. Because intramyocardial vessels make up less than 10 percent of myocardial volume, even with contrast specific imaging methods, myocardial contrast signals are weak compared to those in the LV cavity. Dissolution and disruption of microbubbles by intramural pressure and ultrasound exposure further reduces myocardial contrast. Thus for every contrast method optimal adjustment of the echo machine is crucial to gain maximum sensitivity.

3.3.3.1 Harmonic power Doppler (HPD)

Harmonic power Doppler (HPD) is the current method of choice for myocardial perfusion studies using intravenous infusions of an air based agent such as Levovist (20–24). Harmonic power Doppler is supplied by different manufacturers under different names (*harmonic power angio, loss of correlation imaging*, etc). In the following chapters, the term is used to represent the whole group which function in a technically similar manner. The physics of harmonic power Doppler is described in §1.3.3.2; the specific settings for each system are discussed in §3.6. When using HPD with air-filled contrast agents, the method relies on the detection of bubble echoes which are undergoing rapid change as a result of disruption by the ultrasound beam. It is therefore a high Mechanical Index (MI) method. Since these signals can be obtained from stationary or slowly moving microbubbles, the entire myocardial microcirculation can be detected. The appearance of contrast in the myocardium can easily be visualised since pre-contrast recordings exhibit no HPD in the myocardium (Figure 5). No background subtraction is needed and this is a major advantage over B-mode techniques. Another advantage is the better segmentation of myocardium from the cavities, which is a prerequisite for further quantitative analysis. The signal intensities in the LV cavity and myocardium usually differ by at least 15 dB. The only

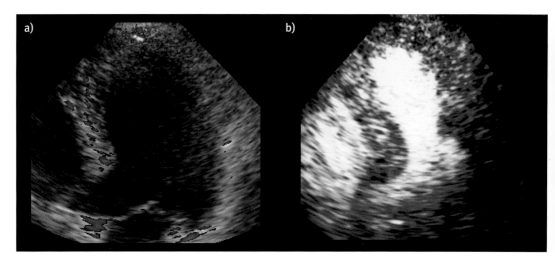

Fig. 9 Power pulse inversion at low MI before (a) and during (b) Definity infusion. Almost no colour is seen within the myocardium at baseline. During infusion intense enhancement is seen within the LV cavity and the entire myocardium. MI = 0.1, framerate = 10 Hz.

Special considerations for myocardial contrast studies

Scanplanes (§3.4.1)	At least two apical views Consider modified scanplanes to improve display of lateral/anterior wall
Triggered imaging (§3.4.2)	Mandatory, except power pulse inversion technique
Contrast administration (§3.5)	Continuous infusion recommended
Machine settings (§3.6)	Different from non-contrast imaging

3.4 Special considerations for myocardial contrast

There are some general requirements which apply to all perfusion imaging studies. These requirements are described here; particular settings for the different imaging techniques will follow in §3.6. Stress testing, reading and interpretation of the findings are common to all imaging modes and are discussed in §3.7–3.9.

3.4.1 Impact of the scanplane

The adjustment of the scanplane has a substantial impact on the success of a myocardial contrast study. First the standard apical planes should be found and optimised as usual (Figure 10). For myocardial contrast studies the grey level in the lateral and anterior wall is a good indicator of how well these segments can be filled with contrast. With regular adjust-

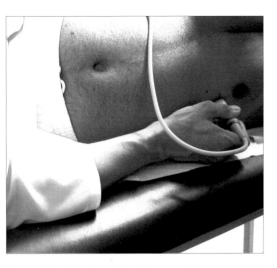

Fig. 10 Positioning the forearm for extended periods when the sonographer is seated to the right of the patient. In order to avoid changing the scanplane during acquisition of triggered images, the forearm is laid on the bed. Scanning without support of the forearm is very strenuous.

ment of the scanplane, the lateral wall (four chamber view) and anterior wall (two chamber view) often have weak or almost no grey within the myocardium. This indicates that local acoustic power is far less than for instance in the septum with high grey levels (Figure 11). The reason for the weaker signals in these segments is attenuation of ultrasound caused by the interposition of pulmonary tissue or ribs. For non-contrast imaging this heterogeneity in grey levels is not a problem as long as endocardial borders are delineated. For contrast studies, however, a reduction in local acoustic power results in reduced or even no contrast signals, which may be misinterpreted as a perfusion defect. Scanplanes should therefore be adjusted in such a way that lateral and anterior walls are displayed with grey myocardium. This can be achieved by slightly changing the scanhead position and moving the lateral or anterior wall further to the centre of the imaging sector (Figure 11). Adjustment of the scanplane should be carried out before injection of contrast. During infusion of contrast the scanplanes should not be changed.

Parasternal views are less suitable for myocardial contrast studies than apical views. Usually the contrast within the right ventricle

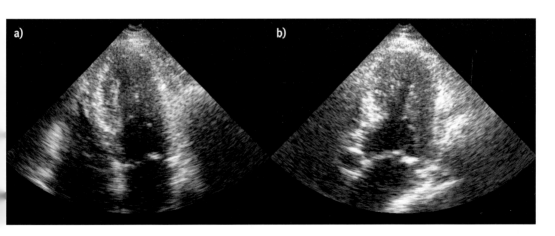

Fig. 11 Adjustment of the four chamber view for a myocardial contrast study. With regular scanning the lateral wall is almost black (a). A slight modification of the scanhead position results in good grey levels in the lateral wall (b).

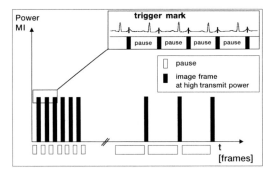

Fig. 12 Triggered imaging: the scanhead only transmits ultrasound for acquisition of single high power frames (black bars), which can be chosen by setting the trigger. The time interval between the acquired frames can be varied by changing the number of cardiac cycles. This schematic illustration demonstrates triggering on each, then on every 7th cardiac cycle.

attenuates the propagation of ultrasound to the deeper parts of the heart, so that inferior and posterior segments cannot be evaluated in many patients. In some patients it is possible to modify the scanplane in such a way that the right ventricle is out of the plane.

3.4.2 Triggered imaging

The disruption of microbubbles by continuous exposure to ultrasound prevents contrast appearing in the myocardium during real-time scanning at high MI. *Intermittent* or *triggered* imaging refers to the interruption of ultrasound exposure between the acquisition of one or more imaging frames (Figure 12). During this interval, the disrupted contrast within the myocardium is replenished and there are again

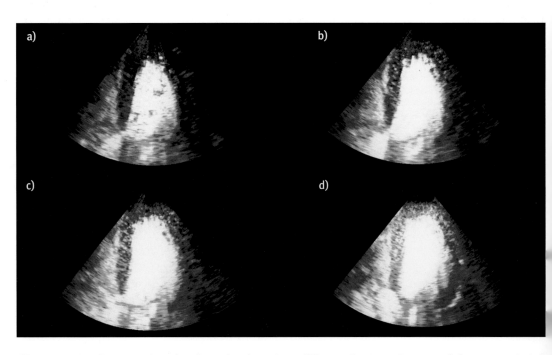

Fig. 13 Harmonic power Doppler, four chamber view, different degrees of myocardial contrast during infusion of Levovist: real time imaging (a), triggered imaging once every cardiac cycle (b), every third cardiac cycle (c) and every 5th cardiac cycle (d).

enough microbubbles to be imaged for the next frame. The frames which are sampled can be selected by trigger markers on the ECG (Figure 12). The sampled image is frozen on the screen of the echo machine until acquisition of the following frame. The introduction of intermittent imaging signalled the initial breakthrough in intravenous myocardial contrast echocardiography (29, 30) and is explained in §1.3.4. In order to replenish the arterial and capillary bed of the myocardium completely, at least 10 seconds are needed. If the percentage of contrast replenishment is plotted against time interval between the imaging frames, an exponential curve is found, the asymptote of which represents full replenishment (see Chapter 4). This means that most replenishment of contrast is found within a period which clinically corresponds to pauses of 5 to 7 cardiac cycles. Therefore trigger rates higher than once every 7th cardiac cycle are usually not necessary.

3.4.2.1 Incremental triggered imaging

It is not possible to predict the optimal trigger intervals in individual patients. The 'best' triggering interval is dependent on cardiac output, dose of echo contrast and the actual attenuation. The recommended protocols therefore include varying trigger intervals with a maximum of one frame every fifth cardiac cycle (Figure 13). In our experience this is long enough to provide a myocardial contrast strong enough to distinguish between perfusion abnormalities in most patients. The incremental pulsing technique is not only suitable for finding the 'best' individual trigger but it can also help quantifying the severity of stenosis.

3.4.2.2 Double or multiple trigger

In double or multiple triggering, the single destruction image is replaced by a short series

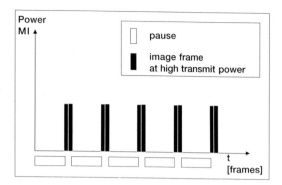

Fig. 14 Double frame triggering: short insonification for acquisition of two frames alternating with periods with no transmission of ultrasound (one or more cardiac cycles).

of imaging frames, acquired in rapid succession (Figure 14). As before, the first frame after the reperfusion interval destroys all of the bubbles in the scanplane and creates the 'perfusion' image. The second and subsequent frames do not show perfusion of the myocardium, but do show cavity flow, as sufficient time has elapsed to allow the faster moving cavity blood to wash new bubbles into the scan plane. Motion artifacts from tissue will also be present in the subsequent frames. One may therefore deduce that only those echoes *present* in the first frame and *absent* in subsequent frames are due to perfusion. This is the main use of multiple triggering. Some systems show the triggered frames side by side, which is especially helpful for interpretation (Figure 15).

3.4.2.3 Flash echo

During intermittent imaging and acquisition of single frames which are frozen until the next frame is sampled, the sonographer does not have control of the scanplane and may lose it because of respiratory or other thoracic motion. An ingenious solution to this problem is to scan continuously in a 'scout' mode during the

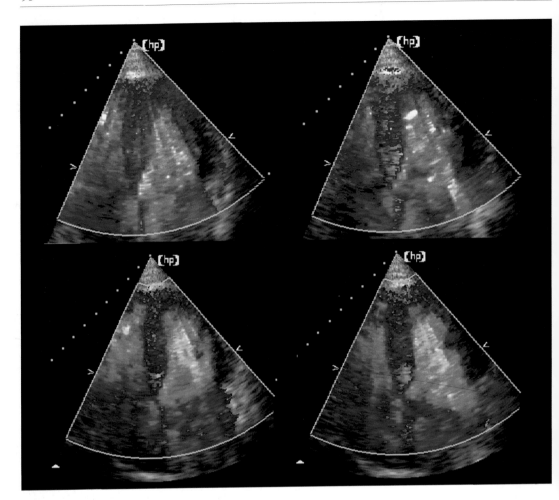

Fig. 15 The double trigger technique: The top panel shows a four chamber view using harmonic Doppler and multiple frame triggering. Every six beats, two high power ultrasound frames are made to disrupt the bubbles within the myocardium. The right panel shows the second frame, where some of the myocardial signal is now absent. This corresponds to bubbles that have been destroyed, an indirect sign of perfusion. The lower two images are from the same patient at a single beat trigger. Imaging every beat does not give enough time to fill the myocardium with bubbles. Therefore, the coloured myocardium is not a sign of perfusion. Persistence of myocardial harmonic power Doppler signals in the second frame suggests motion artifact rather than perfusion.
Courtesy of J Luis Zamorano, University of Madrid, Spain

interval with low emission power (MI < 0.2) which does not disrupt the bubbles (Figure 16). With low MI harmonic imaging, contrast can be displayed in the cavities but not in the myocardium; cardiac structures can be displayed for correction of the scanplane if the patient breathes or moves. Destruction frames at high MI are triggered as before, creating the perfusion image. Multiple triggering may also be used.

3.4.2.4 Power pulse inversion flash echo

The superior sensitivity of power pulse inversion

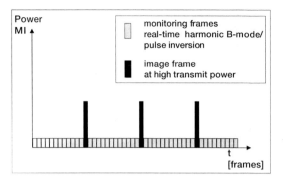

Fig. 16 Flash imaging: continuous scanning with low transmit power using low transmit power is performed to adjust the scanplane without display of myocardial contrast. Single frames are acquired with high transmit power to image myocardial contrast. The power pulse inversion method uses the same sequence of frames allowing display of myocardial contrast signals in real-time at low transmit power. Single or multiple periods of insonification may be used to destroy the myocardial microbubbles and to assess myocardial contrast replenishment.

(PPI) in detecting bubbles at low MI means that intermittent imaging is not needed for power pulse inversion to achieve display of myocardial contrast, because low transmit power results in only minor destruction of microbubbles. However, even with PPI, triggering may still provide a benefit. During continuous imaging of perfusion at low MI, a single high power frame may be used to disrupt the contrast agent within the myocardial tissue and then to assess reperfusion in real-time (see §4.2.3.3). Real time dynamics of myocardial contrast replenishment provides additional information to the steady signal intensities seen during infusion.

3.4.2.5 Systolic versus diastolic trigger

Contrast imaging is often improved when frames are sampled during systole rather than during diastole. The small systolic cavity causes less attenuation compared to diastole and the thickened myocardium facilitates further quantitative analysis, for instance by allowing regions of interest to be positioned without touching the cavity. Moreover, the myocardium moves to the centre of the imaging sector where sensitivity to contrast is better than in the lateral sectors of the imaging field. However, myocardial blood flow is highest during diastole and especially subendocardial vessels are squeezed during systole. Since myocardial contrast echo evaluates the blood volume and the replenishment which takes several cardiac cycles, it is probably irrelevant which portion of the cardiac cycle is chosen for data acquisition. Positioning the trigger point is easy with harmonic B-mode, where just the frame at the top of T-wave should be selected. In power Doppler, wall motion artifacts may be present, requiring the sonographer to take special measures to suppress these artifacts or look for other frames with fewer artifacts (for specific suggestions see §3.6.1.1).

3.5 Choice of agent and method of administration

3.5.1 Continuous infusion versus bolus injection

Until recently, bolus injections have been widely used for myocardial contrast echo. They still may be used for a rest study in acute transmural myocardial infarction, providing qualitative information as to whether there is a perfusion defect or reperfusion. For all other indications, the contrast agent should be administered as an infusion (Figure 17, 18). Although administration by bolus saves some time, there are a number of disadvantages,

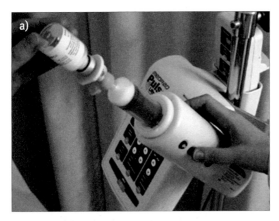
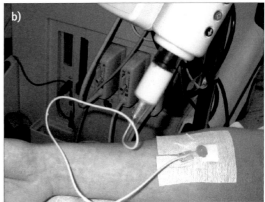

Fig. 17 Infusion of Levovist for myocardial contrast echocardiography. A PULSAR system (Medrad Inc.) filled with two vials of 4 g Levovist (a) with a short tube connected with the venous cannula in a cubital vein (b).

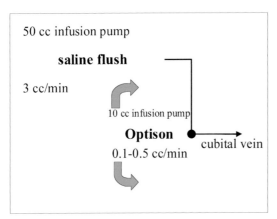
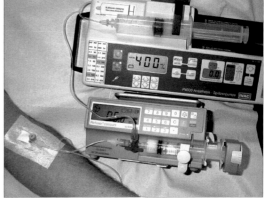

Fig. 18 Set-up for infusion of undiluted perfluorocarbon agents. The undiluted agent is infused at low speed, a saline infusion at high speed prevents settlement of the microbbubbles within the tubes and the vein. This allows continuous infusion of Optison, but agitating the pump is necessary during infusion (left). For Definity this set-up is recommended only for real-time perfusion imaging, but agitation is not necessary (right).

most notably the comparatively short time for data acquisition, frequent artifacts and greatly reduced ability to quantify the resulting data. Wei *et al.* offer the following reasons for using an infusion (31, 32):

1. It is relatively easy to adjust the dose of contrast agent to the patient's particular imaging conditions.
2. Blooming and contrast shadowing, regular occurrences with administration by bolus, can be considerably reduced by titrating the infusion rate for each individual.
3. Loosing the scanplane – not an uncommon occurrence in intermittent imaging – does not result in loss of the study. Recordings can be repeated under compar-

able conditions or additional, modified planes can be imaged.
4. The infusion can be started or modified by the same person who is performing the ultrasound recordings. Repeated administrations of bolus usually require an extra pair of hands.
5. A simple quantification of myocardial contrast effect can only be achieved by using a stable contrast infusion.

3.5.2 Preparation of contrast infusion

For infusion of Levovist, a venous line should be introduced into a cubital vein. For other agents and vasodilator stress, forearm veins can be used. Preparation of the contrast agent should not begin before the pre-contrast scanning has shown that the patient is suitable for a myocardial contrast study (good image quality, no contraindications). When harmonic power Doppler is used, the triggered frames should show no wall motion artifacts and good 'spontaneous contrast' in the LV cavity.

3.5.3 Adjustment of infusion rate

Optimisation of infusion rate is performed by visual evaluation of contrast intensities in the apical and basal segments using triggered imaging (one frame every 5th beat is best to begin

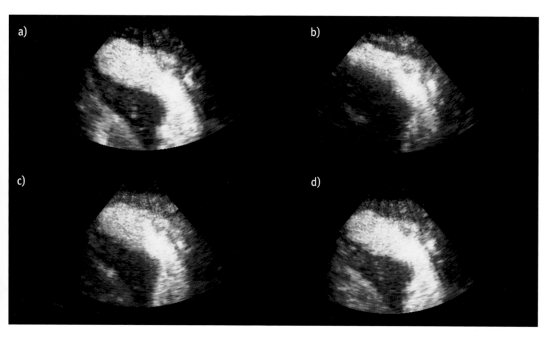

Fig. 19 Impact of the infusion rate on the display of myocardial contrast (harmonic power Doppler, modified four chamber view with optimal display of the lateral wall, infusion of Levovist). a) Dose too low, full opacification of LV, but weak contrast signals within the myocardium. b) Dose too high, contrast shadowing, strong signals in the nearfield but no signals at greater depth. c) Dose too low, septum signal intensities are low compared to the lateral wall suggesting a perfusion deficit. d) Optimal dose with similar signal intensities in septum and lateral wall.

Dosing of ultrasound contrast agents for myocardial perfusion

Contrast agent	Contents of vial	Dilution	Required number of vials	Cannula size	Loading bolus	Initial infusion rate
Levovist	4 g granulate	add water to 400 mg/ml	2 vials	18 gauge	2 ml	1.5–5 ml/min*
Optison**	Suspension for injection	undiluted (3 ml vial)	1 vial	20 gauge	0.3 ml	7 ml/h
Definity	Suspension for injection (1.3 ml vial)	1.3 ml in 50 ml saline	1 vial	18–20 gauge	0.5 ml	6 ml/min

* Depending on ultrasound imaging system
** Not stable in a regular infusion pump, special set-up necessary (Figure 18) (33)

with). Weak signals in the entire myocardium indicate underdosing of contrast (Figure 19). An optimal infusion results in homogeneous contrast enhancement in the apical and basal segments. In this situation cavity contrast saturates and strong cavity signals can be seen within the left atrium as well as the left ventricle. Intense signals in the nearfield but weak or absent signals at a greater depth indicate contrast shadowing: the infusion rate should be reduced. Guidelines as to how to adjust the infusion rate for some different agents are listed in the Table. Because of the time needed to reach a steady state, adjustment of dose should not be performed in intervals of less than one minute.

contrast echo some parameters which are not touched in routine B-mode and Doppler echocardiography become crucial. The trainee in myocardial contrast echo must learn how to manipulate some controls of the echo machine which he or she has never used before. Careful adjustment is necessary, as even minor deviations from the optimal setting may result in a dramatic reduction in sensitivity. First, initial settings are given which may be stored as scanner 'presets'. Next, we provide guidelines for optimising settings for each individual patient's conditions. This adjustment of instrument controls is performed before infusion of contrast, so that during the contrast infusion itself no further changes are usually necessary.

3.6 Instrument settings

For successful studies correct adjustment of the imaging system to the specific acoustic properties of the contrast agent is essential. In

3.6.1 Harmonic power Doppler

In harmonic power Doppler, the aim is to achieve complete disruption of the contrast agent in the myocardium and to display the power Doppler signal without also displaying tissue motion artifact. The most important machine settings are listed below. Please note that the effect of machine settings varies with individual machine architecture. The recommendations that follow are for initial settings and should be read in conjunction with those suggested by the manufacturer.

3.6.1.1 Setting the trigger point

During spontaneous respiration the trigger point is set at the top of the T-wave and intermittent imaging is performed with one frame each cardiac cycle. After recording of several cardiac frames in triggered mode, a visual check should be made as to whether wall motion artifacts are superimposed on the myocardium (Figure 20). It is essential that no colour signals should be visible within the myocardium before injection of contrast. Within the LV cavity there may be some spontaneous harmonic power Doppler contrast throughout the entire cardiac cycle. Wall motion artifacts must be evaluated during triggered imaging, as artifacts in continuous imaging will be different.

If wall motion artifacts are visible, the following manoeuvres may be undertaken:

1. *Changing the trigger point* by advancing or delaying in single increments. This will be effective in most patients. If no systolic frame can be found without wall motion artifacts, diastolic triggering can be set with a trigger shortly before the onset of the P-wave.

2. *Controlled breathing or breathold.* In patients with wall motion artifacts induced by respiratory movements, holding the breath can be tolerated only for frames with a high trigger rate. For longer trigger intervals 'controlled breathing' is recommended: the patient is asked to breathe shallowly and arrest inspiration when the imaging frame is obtained. The patient should have some practice with this technique before baseline and contrast recordings are performed.

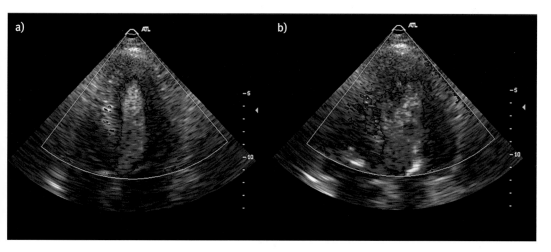

Fig. 20 Selection of the trigger position for intermittent imaging: four chamber view, two consecutive frames acquired during baseline: a) shows optimal trigger point with no wall motion artifacts, b) is not useful because of wall motion artifacts in the lateral wall and the septum. Note intracavitary harmonic power Doppler signals in both frames.

3. *Increasing the PRF.* By reducing the period between, this reduces motion artifact. It also reduces sensitivity to the contrast agent.

4. *Increasing wall filter setting.* This also eliminates some of the contrast signal, so should be used carefully.

5. *Increasing the colour threshold.* This is a somewhat perilous measure that will eliminate any of the contrast signal whose strength is below that of the moving tissue. Not recommended!

6. *Decreasing the colour gain.* A last resort, which can often reduce sensitivity to the contrast agent to the point that it will not be seen on infusion. If a gain adjustment must be made, a satisfactory level to eliminate artifact should be established before contrast, but

Harmonic power Doppler perfusion studies: settings

Initial settings for all systems (preset):

Scanhead	Lowest frequency
Transmit power	Mechanical Index (MI) > 1.2
Receive gain	Default
Display-Mode	Standard monochromatic map
Dynamic range	Maximum
Persistence	Disabled
Line density	Lowest value
Sensitivity	Medium
Wall filter	High
PRF	1500 kHz (Optison/Definity), 2500 kHz (Levovist)

Individual adjustment of instrument controls:

Scanplane	Conventional planes
	Optimise in tissue harmonic mode (see text) then reduce receive gain for tissue harmonic
Imaging field	Adjust box so that the entire LV-myocardium is included
Focus	Below mitral valve (apical planes),
	Below posterior wall (parasternal view)
	HP system: move towards apex if apical defect present
Trigger	Systole (peak of T-wave)
	Double trigger, if available
	Once every cardiac cycle (increase during infusion of contrast)
	Carefully adjust to avoid wall motion artifacts (see text)

implemented only after arrival of the contrast, when its effect on the study can be seen.

If double frame acquisition is available, both consecutive frames should be checked for wall motion artifacts, as they are acquired at slightly different points in the cardiac cycle.

3.6.2 Harmonic B-mode

Harmonic B-mode may be used if the available instrument does not provide harmonic power Doppler or if the offline subtraction method has been chosen. Harmonic response increases with transmit intensity of ultrasound, so a high MI is recommended (see Table). The user should be prepared, however, to see strong pre-contrast echoes from tissue harmonics. In fact, a good

Harmonic B-mode for myocardial perfusion: settings

Initial settings for all systems (preset):

Scanhead	Lowest frequency
Transmit power	Mechanical index (MI) > 1.2
Receive gain	Default
Compression	None
Dynamic range	Maximum
Persistence	Disabled
Line density	Lowest value

Individual adjustment of instrument controls:

Scanplanes	Find conventional planes then reduce receive gain (see text)
Focus	Below mitral valve (apical planes), Below posterior wall (parasternal view)
Transmit power	Reduce initial level if apical defect or swirling is seen. Increase MI if global contrast is too weak
Receive gain	May be reduced slightly to suppress myocardial tissue echo
TGC	As in standard imaging
Lateral gain (HP)	As in non-contrast imaging
Trigger	Systole (peak of T-wave). Once every cardiac cycle (increase during infusion of contrast)

Understanding machine settings for harmonic power Doppler perfusion studies

Control	Setting	Comments
Mode	Harmonic power angio	Also known as: *coded harmonic angio; colour power angio; harmonic power Doppler.*
Transducer frequency	Lowest, eg 1.5/3.0 MHz	Lower frequencies give better bubble disruption and hence sensitivity, but slightly poorer resolution.
Output power (MI)	High: MI > 1.0	High MI is essential for bubble disruption. Usually the maximum is best.
Colour box size/position	Embrace entire myocardium of interest	MI reduces at edges of sector, making imaging there less reliable.
Focus	Level of mitral valve	Focus affects uniformity of exposure conditions in image. With some systems (eg HP Sonos 5500), it is necessary to move focus to apex to see perfusion there.
Pulse repetition frequency (PRF)	2.5–4.0kHz	Also known as: *Doppler scale.* Highest possible. Lower PRF increases sensitivity to both contrast but also tissue motion. Air agents (eg Levovist) work better at high PRF than perfluorocarbon agents (eg Optison or Definity).
Trigger	Mid T-wave (initial setting)	Note that trigger often affects MI. Adjust trigger to minimise motion artifacts and adjust other controls with trigger active.
Frames	2–4	This controls the number of frames acquired at each trigger. The first frame shows contrast combined with artifacts, subsequent frames show artifacts only.
Dual display	On (if available)	With multiframe trigger, a dual image display showing first and a subsequent frame can help interpretation of contrast perfusion study.
Colour gain	Decrease to the point that motion artifacts are just visible in pre-contrast image	Adjust gain last, after trigger, PRF, filter and other colour settings have been adjusted to minimise motion artifact.
B-mode gain	Sufficient to see endocardium	Excessively high B-mode gain can cause grey to overwrite colour in image.

Control	Setting	Comments
Colour priority	Maximum	Also known as: *Angio priority*. Forces colour to overwrite grey level in image.
Colour threshold	Minimum	Removes low level contrast signals: must be set to zero
Line density	Minimum	Reducing line density limits inadvertent bubble destruction (that is, bubble destruction that does not contribute to the image). Increasing frame rate setting may also decrease line density.
Frame rate	Medium – High	Higher frame rates may decrease line density
Persistence	Zero	Also known as: *frame averaging*. Contrast signals are typically present in a single frame. Averaging may reduce their value.
Ensemble length	Medium – High (8 pulses)	Also known as: *Doppler sensitivity, packet length*. This determines the number of pulses sent along each scan line. A high number improves both bubble disruption rate and sensitivity to the agent. Lower settings can be used for Levovist.
Dynamic range	High	Too low dynamic range will create an 'on/off' display of colour; too high will increase background noise and blooming from the cavity
Wall Filter	Medium – Low	Also known as: *low velocity reject*. Eliminates signals from slowly moving structures such as tissue. At too high a level, will also reject contrast echoes. Use the lowest setting possible, while still eliminating motion artifact from tissue.

way to predict whether adequate contrast signals will be obtained in the lateral wall is to check whether clear tissue harmonic echoes can be seen in these areas. Thus one first ensures that there is a good tissue harmonic echo using a normal gain setting, after which the receive gain is reduced in readiness for the contrast study. At baseline the myocardium should be almost black and only the endocardial borders should be visible.

As with power Doppler, the position of the transmit focus and the line density affect bubble disruption. Reduction of line density compared to that used for non-contrast imaging and placing the focus below the mitral valve helps to make insonation more homogeneous. Dynamic range should be as high as possible to ensure that small changes in contrast signals are not overlooked. Compression and other forms of nonlinear processing which

Pulse inversion imaging for myocardial perfusion: settings

Initial settings for all systems (preset):

Transmit power	Mechanical Index (MI) = 0.3 for triggered imaging
Receive gain	Default
Compression	None
Dynamic range	Maximum
Persistence	Disabled
Line density	Regular

Individual adjustment of instrument controls:

Scanplanes	Corresponding to conventional planes.
	Optimise before injection of contrast (see text), then reduce receive gain
Focus	Below mitral valve (apical planes),
	Below posterior wall (parasternal view)
Receive gain	Adjust to be just above the noise level
TGC	As in standard imaging
Trigger	Systole (peak of T-wave)
	Once every cardiac cycle (increase during infusion of contrast)
	Adjust to reduce motion artifact

enhance the display of diagnostic information in non-contrast echocardiography serve only to corrupt the interpretation of regional myocardial perfusion echoes. Therefore no compression should be used for myocardial contrast echo. Positioning of the trigger is easy with harmonic B-mode and the double trigger (frame) technique is not required to check for artifacts. However, the double frame technique may be used for subtraction during contrast infusion.

3.6.3 Pulse inversion imaging

Similar adjustments are necessary for the pulse inversion method as for harmonic B-mode. To date, there is limited experience with this method, so the recommendations listed in the Table are preliminary. The pulse inversion method has a remarkable sensitivity for contrast at low transmit power settings and is much more effective than harmonic power Doppler or harmonic B-mode at low MI. It is therefore recommended to work with lower MIs with pulse inversion imaging than with harmonic B-mode, as the reduction in tissue harmonic improves myocardial perfusion contrast. With lower MI, a lower infusion rate may also be more effective. For quantitative analysis, which should be the aim of every myocardial contrast study, triggered imaging is still as necessary as it is with the other imaging methods. With triggered imaging the contrast effect increases with increasing transmit power. Spatial resolution is much better with pulse inversion than with power Doppler or harmonic B-mode. The potential problem of motion artifact in greyscale pulse inversion imaging means that special attention should be paid to the trigger point and to the pulse repetition frequency, as with harmonic power Doppler. In some systems, increasing the pulse repetition frequency can be achieved simply by increasing the framerate, which will tend to reduce motion artifact at the expense of some loss of sensitivity to the agent.

Power pulse inversion for real-time myocardial perfusion: settings

Initial settings for all systems (preset):

Transmit power	Mechanical index (MI) = 0.15
PRF	2500 Hz
Dynamic range	Low
Sensitivity	Medium
Persistence	Disabled
Line density	Low (increases frame rate)
Penetration depth	12.7 cm
Focus	10 cm
Receive gain	Default

Individual adjustment of instrument controls:

Transmit power	Good window : MI = 0.09–0.11
	Moderate window: MI = 0.11–0.14
Scanplanes	Corresponding to conventional planes
	optimise before injection of contrast (see text)
TGC	Depth 1 ~ 30 optimise to suppress tissue harmonics
	Depth 2 > 50 optimise to suppress tissue harmonics
	Depth 3–8 maximum
Trigger*	Optional – peak of the R wave
	Once every 15th cardiac cycle
	Double frame (MI = 0.5)

* can be used to destroy microbubbles in myocardium for real-time destruction-reperfusion measurement (see §4.2.3)

3.6.4 Power pulse inversion

This is the only method which currently allows real-time perfusion imaging. Preliminary settings are listed in the Table. In practice, 'real-time' means frame rates of up to about 26 Hz. Very low transmit power (MI = 0.09–0.15) is the essential prerequisite for visualising myocardial contrast in real-time. With current technology effective myocardial contrast can only be achieved with perfluorocarbon agents. Higher doses are needed: bolus injections of 0.5–1.0 ml of Optison or infusion rates of 0.5 ml/min provide good myocardial contrast. Single or double frames with high transmit power may be used to destroy the microbubbles within the myocardium and to assess re-plenishment in real-time (see §4.2.3.3). No triggering is necessary.

3.7. Image acquisition

As with conventional stress echocardiography, all recordings should be digitally stored and analysed offline. Capabilities for digital image storage are provided in all harmonic echo machines, using direct connection to a DICOM network or by magneto-optical (MO) discs. Before each contrast study, a check must be made to see whether there is enough space to store the study. Videotape is a useful backup and also forms a continuous record. During data acquisition shallow breathing is recommended. Holding the breath is not useful for triggered imaging, because many cardiac patients are unable to do so for sufficiently long to cover several frames at long trigger intervals. It usually takes at least two minutes before the myocardial microbubble concentration has reached a steady state. Thus contrast recordings should be started three minutes after contrast infusion has been initiated (Figure 21). The recommended recordings for all imaging modalities except power pulse inversion imaging are shown in the Table.

Power pulse inversion imaging can be performed in real-time. At least 5 cardiac cycles should be sampled in each view. Breatholding is often useful to obtain reproducible consecutive cycles.

Recommended image files to document a myocardial contrast study

Baseline	Rest	Stress
• four chamber view • two chamber view • long axis	• four chamber view • two chamber view • long axis	• four chamber view • two chamber view • long axis

- Each file should include at least 5 frames, triggered 1:1, 1:3 and 1:5.
- With real-time imaging at least 3 cardiac cycles should be recorded, followed by the destruction bursts and the variable period of myocardial contrast replenishment which is completed within 10 cardiac cycles.
- Baseline recordings are necessary in PPI and HPD to prove, that tissue harmonics and wall motion harmonics are eliminated. With B-mode harmonic and pulse inversion imaging baseline recordings are needed for background subtraction.

3.8 Stress testing during myocardial contrast echo

3.8.1 Exercise and dobutamine stress

During myocardial contrast echo, stress can be performed with any of the available methods, though the special imaging conditions make pharmacological stress more suitable. Exercise stress (exercise or treadmill) provides the greatest myocardial oxygen consumption compared to other methods (10). However, scanning during and after exercise is difficult because of increased respiratory and cardiac motion. At peak stress it is sometimes a problem to keep or reproduce the same scanplane, because the patient may be unable to hold his or her breath. Because myocardial contrast echo requires recording a series of consecutive triggered frames, physical exercise is a challenging procedure for the echocardiographer. With pulse inversion imaging or harmonic power Doppler, wall motion artifacts are accentuated following an increase in heart rate and inotropic state leading to further reduction of image quality. Finally, the need to adjust the trigger point to the varying heart rate further complicates the method.

Dobutamine infusion only slightly reduces these difficulties. At peak stress there are problems similar to those found during physical exercise, where the enhanced cardiac and respiratory motion limits scanning, particularly with harmonic power Doppler and pulse inversion. Thus vasodilator stress is our method of choice for myocardial stress contrast echocardiography.

3.8.2 Vasodilator stress

During dipyridamole and adenosine infusion the changes in heart rate are moderate and the inotropic state is not altered significantly. As a result, oxygen consumption is not increased. Ischemia only develops with additional horizontal or vertical steal (Figure 22), which is found in up to 50 percent of patients with sig-

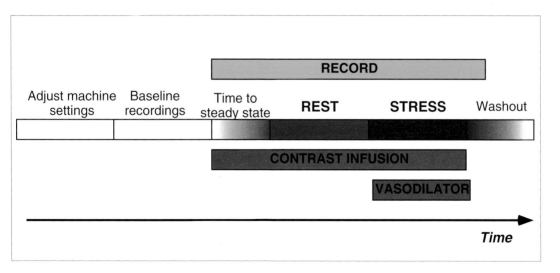

Fig. 21 Protocol for resting and stress studies.

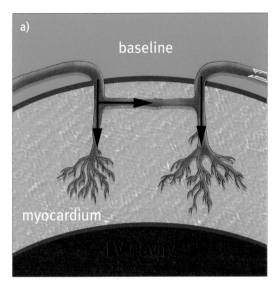 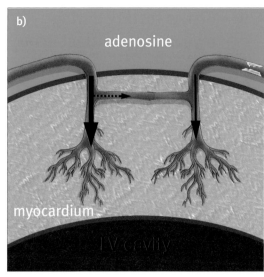

Fig. 22 Effects of adenosine on intramyocardial vessels in normal epicardial coronary arteries and in the presence of a stenosis. At baseline (a) the blood flow in the perfusion bed of the stenosed coronary artery is not different from areas without stenoses due to maximal dilatation of the arterioles and collateral flow. With adenosine (b) arteriolar resistance decreases in the normally perfused territory resulting in a 3- to 4-fold increase of blood flow in the normal myocardium. In the presence of a significant stenosis blood flow does not increase, but may decrease due to reduced collateral flow (*steal* phenomenon).

nificant stenoses. Only these patients develop wall motion abnormalities. Thus wall motion abnormalities are found less frequently with vasodilator stress than with exercise or dobutamine. However, blood flow in the perfusion bed supplied by a significantly stenosed artery increases only marginally (or decreases when steal phenomena develop) compared to the three to four fold increase in areas supplied by non-stenotic arteries, and a perfusion mismatch can be displayed with high sensitivity (34, 35).

The myocardial segments not affected by coronary artery stenosis will show an increase in signal intensities corresponding to their normal flow reserve whereas hypoperfused areas will show no increase in signal intensities or even a decrease due to a steal. Evaluation of vasodilator stress images can be performed by visual judgement or by using post-processing and quantitative analysis (see §4.2). Since vasodilator stress is not widely used for conventional stress echocardiography, the dose regimen and side effects and contraindications are reviewed in the Tables. Side-effects are common, particularly for adenosine stress, but they are benign. Dipyridamole and adenosine have extra-cardiac effects which limit scanning during infusion of contrast. The most important is dyspnea which causes deep breathing and threatens loss of the imaging plane. The patient must be informed about this phenomenon before starting the adenosine infusion. Many patients can tolerate the discomfort if they are informed before the examination.

Choosing a stress modality for harmonic power Doppler

	Ease of scanning	Induced ischemia	Modality of choice
Physical exercise	difficult	needed	2 D harmonic PPI
Dobutamine	difficult	needed	2 D harmonic PPI
Dipyridamole	easier	not necessary	all modalities
Adenosine	easier	not necessary	all modalities

3.8.3 Combined assessment of wall motion and myocardial perfusion

Myocardial contrast echocardiography can be performed in conjunction with a routine stress echo protocol for wall motion analysis (see §3.3.1). With real-time perfusion imaging simultaneous assessment of perfusion and wall motion is possible using a constant infusion of contrast (Figure 23). With triggered imaging contrast infusion should be confined to MCE recordings for two reasons: contrast is not needed for left ventricular opacification (LVO) because good acoustic windows are recommended for perfusion studies. Furthermore, the doses for MCE using triggerd imaging are lower than for real-time LVO studies and

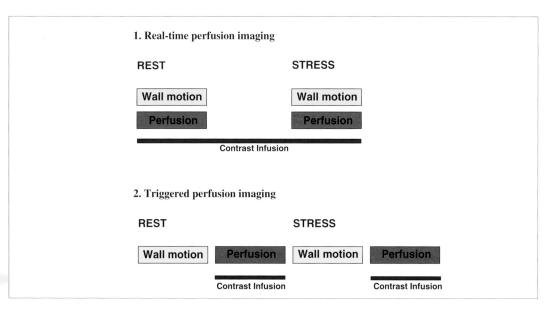

Fig. 23 How to integrate an MCE study using triggered imaging into a routine stress echo protocol for wall motion analysis. With adequate baseline images contrast infusion can be confined to MCE recordings.

adjusting infusion speeds to LVO or MCE is difficult with the time constraints of a stress test.

3.9 Reading myocardial contrast echocardiograms

Reading MCE studies involves steps which are similar to those of a regular stress echo for evaluation of LV wall motion, which may parallel a perfusion study. In each view the segments defined by the American Society of Echocardiography (ASE) are evaluated and the corresponding segments at rest and during stress are compared. Reading and interpretation of perfusion studies needs to be performed offline. Visual assessment of perfusion, however, is mandatory during the stress phase of the contrast study: if perfusion defects develop under stress, the stress should be stopped. The following guidelines for reading and interpretation apply to all imaging techniques. The evaluation of triggered images is in principle not different to that of images made with real-time perfusion imaging. There are several ways to deal with the stored recordings:
- Visual judgement of original single frames and cine loops,
- Visual judgement of post-processed images,
- Quantitative analysis of original or postprocessed images

Original recordings can be used for harmonic power Doppler and power pulse inversion, whereas evaluation of recordings obtained with harmonic B-mode is more difficult. When using a greyscale technique at high MI, the contrast signals need to be separated from the tissue harmonic signals present at baseline. Because this is so difficult to appreciate subjectively from the compressed grey levels seen on the screen, background subtraction and colour coding must be applied before visual judgement is attempted from harmonic B-mode recordings.

3.9.1 Visual assessment of unprocessed recordings

Visual assessment is practicable with power Doppler and power pulse inversion recordings. High MI greyscale images should not be assessed in this way. However, once software tools for background subtraction and colour coding of the myocardial contrast signals have been applied, visual judgement of processed greyscale images uses the same criteria as those for the assessment of unprocessed power Doppler images. Visual judgement mainly relies on the signal intensities of myocardial contrast, which reflects relative myocardial blood volume. In order to get an idea of myocardial blood flow, one needs to evaluate the changes in the signal intensities with time. A very rough estimate of flow is provided by the time needed to achieve visible myocardial

Visual grading of myocardial contrast: separate scores for each of the six ASE myocardial segments of the scanplane	
0	No contrast enhancement
1	Poor contrast enhancement, incomplete filling of segment
2	Moderate contrast enhancement, complete filling
3	Strong contrast enhancement
X	Unsuccessful (artifacts, attenuation, blooming, etc)

contrast following the disruption of myocardial contrast by high power frames (36). With the power pulse inversion method this replenishment can be recorded in real-time. Using the other methods and triggered imaging, one can determine lowest trigger interval at which myocardial contrast becomes visible.

3.9.1.1 Normal perfusion

The dose regimen and machine settings listed in §3.6 provide moderate or strong contrast enhancement at the longer trigger intervals (1:3–1:5). At shorter intervals (1:1–1:3), the contrast pattern is patchy or reticular, representing the larger intramyocardial vessels. More homogeneous opacification is found with intervals above 1:3 (Figure 24). With optimal display, myocardial contrast involves the entire myocardial thickness (Figures 25, 26). Isolated epicardial contrast is caused by display of epicardial vessels and may be found during wash-in of contrast following a bolus injection but not during infusion and triggered imaging. In power Doppler mode, isolated epicardial colour signals represent wall motion artifacts rather than vascular contrast (see §3.11.4).

Before MCE studies are evaluated, the reader should judge the corresponding scanplanes for wall motion. At rest all segments without wall motion abnormalities should show contrast enhancement. Missing or incomplete myocardial contrast in a normally contracting muscle is an artifact! Incomplete myocardial contrast enhancement may often be found in normals – particularly in the basal segments. These basal dropouts represent attenuation rather than real perfusion defects – especially when the defect does not end in the myocardium. During stress these segments often fill in. Coronary stenoses usually involve mid and apical segments, so that isolated basal defects seem to have only minor clinical impact.

The variation of exposure to transmitted ultrasound in different parts of the image should always be taken into account in a visual

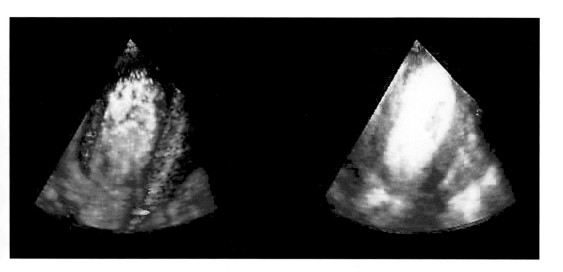

Fig. 24 Example of successful visualisation of all segments in modified four chamber view during Levovist infusion.

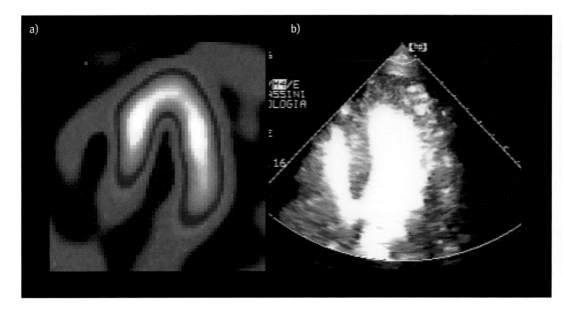

Fig. 25 Normal perfusion: SPECT, horizontal axis (a) and harmonic power Doppler, four chamber view (b).
Courtesy of Francesco Gentile, University of Milan, Italy

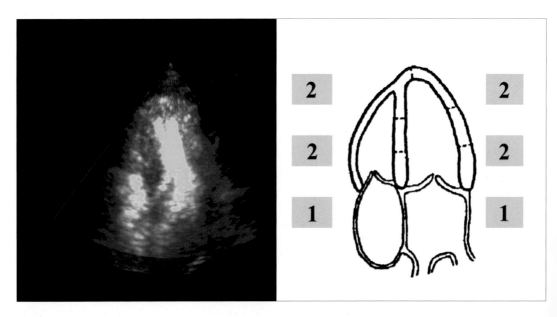

Fig. 26 Harmonic power Doppler, four chamber view, Optison infusion. Two frames showing normal findings with excellent delineation of cavity from myocardial signals. Note the intense spots within the myocardium which represent intramyocardial vessels. In the right frame the myocardial contrast scores of the six segments are shown.
Courtesy of Joanne Sandelski and Steve Feinstein, Rush University, Chicago IL, USA

assessment. When perfusion is normal, signals of varying intensity are found in the individual myocardial segments (Figures 26, 27). This is because the effective mechanical index is not the same at all points in the image plane. In lateral regions, the transducer transmits less intense pulses; in deep regions attenuation reduces the intensity progressively (Figure 28).

Dropouts in the entire lateral wall (four chamber view) and the anterior wall (two chamber view) should be rare when the imaging guidelines are followed. If lateral or anterior dropouts cannot be eliminated, the diagnostic value of an MCE study is limited. However, in some circumstances, it is not necessary to achieve good contrast signals in the entire myocardium. For instance, in a perfusion study for the assessment of the significance of an LAD stenosis, lateral dropout can be tolerated.

During stress an increase in myocardial signal intensity is observed. Due to an increase of myocardial blood flow, myocardial opacification is seen at lower trigger intervals than in the rest study. With real-time imaging, a corresponding reduction of contrast replenishment time is found. At rest it usually takes three or more cardiac cycles to fill the myocardium,

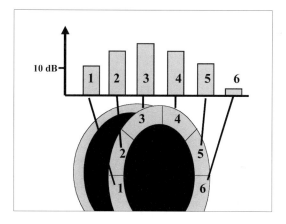

Fig. 27 Mean Doppler power in patients with normal myocardial perfusion (four chamber view): note the differences between the myocardial segments during infusion of Levovist.

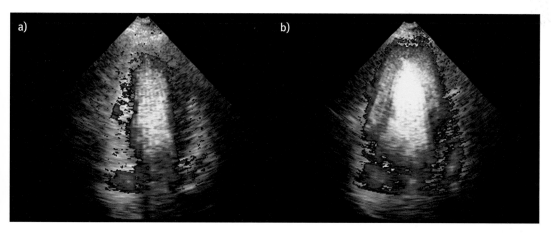

Fig. 28 Normal perfusion, harmonic power Doppler, two chamber view (infusion of Levovist). a) shows early LV filling during wash-in of contrast with some wall motion artifacts in the inferior wall. Note the lower grey signal intensities in the anterior wall compared to the inferior wall because of lower local acoustic power. With optimised dosing of contrast infusion (b), intense contrast signals are found in the entire inferior wall. The display of contrast in the anterior wall is excellent in the apical and mid segments but not in the basal segment.
Courtesy of Gerd P Meyer, University of Hanover, Germany

whereas myocardial contrast is seen within a single cardiac cycle during adenosine infusion.

A side-by-side display of the baseline and stress frames or loops is recommended when reading perfusion stress studies. The best approach for visual assessment is the comparison of the same segments at baseline and during stress. If weak or no signals are seen in a segment, one should check for echoes in the deeper-lying segments. With septal and inferior defects, the opposite wall can also be compared. Note that this procedure does not work in reverse. If no strong signals are detectable in the compared segments, the diagnosis of a perfusion defect is not safe.

3.9.1.2 Perfusion defect

To date, myocardial scintigraphy has been the only clinical method to image myocardial perfusion. Myocardial contrast echocardiography aims to replace scintigraphic techniques and partly uses the same kind of reading. However, display of myocardial perfusion is different for the two modalities. Often scintigraphic defects do not match the size of MCE defects. The poor spatial resolution and the special processing of myocardial scintigraphy result in perfusion deficits which usually extend over the entire thickness of the LV wall. It is known, though, that perfusion abnormalities often involve subendocardial layers with preserved flow in subepicardial layers. Due to its better spatial resolution, MCE has provided for the first time display of subendocardial ischemia (Figure 29). It too is capable of showing patchy and transmural patterns of perfusion defects, however (Figure 30).

As with myocardial scintigraphy, perfusion defects with contrast echo are classified as fixed or reversible. A fixed defect is marked by a relative decrease in signal intensity compared to the adjacent myocardium, visible at rest and during exercise. It may be subendocardial or transmural. The apparent degree of a perfusion defect depends on the amount of contrast present in the vessels of normally perfused myocardium compared to the vessels within the hypoperfused area. Even in a scar after a transmural infarction, it will be seen that some vessels are visible. High amounts of contrast within these vessels may cause intense signals and even blooming which may obscure the visual delineation of the hypoperfused areas. Since the amount of myocardial contrast is dependent on the trigger interval and the infusion rate of the contrast agent, the display of a perfusion deficit is variable (Figure 31). Perfusion defects may decrease or even disappear with increasing contrast dose or trigger interval! This is particularly true for harmonic power Doppler studies where blooming is more evident than with the other imaging modalities. Careful evaluation of all images sampled at different trigger intervals is mandatory: frames with blooming or saturation must not be used for evaluation. Due to these limitations, the absolute size of a perfusion defect should not be estimated. It is sufficient to specify the segments in which contrast patterns look abnormal.

Reversible defects appear normal at rest but become visible during stress, where a marked increase of signal intensity is observed in normal myocardium, compared to a slight increase or even a decrease in the defect area. Thus, during peak stress reversible defects show a relative decrease in signal intensity compared to adjacent normal myocardium. Usually the delineation is enhanced at lower trigger intervals, when normally perfused tissue exhibits a moderate or strong contrast enhancement. The

Perfusion Imaging 117

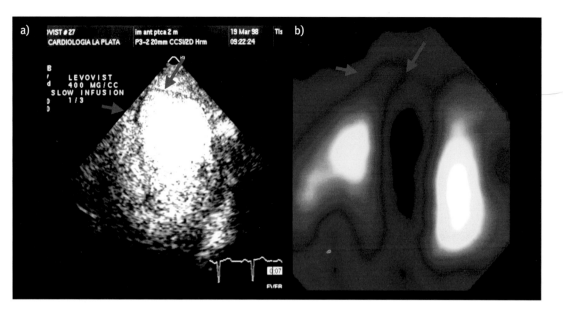

Fig. 29 Harmonic B-mode, four chamber view, continuous infusion of Levovist, post apical myocardial infarction. a) Subendocardial perfusion defect. b) Transmural defect in corresponding plane of Thallium SPECT at rest.
Courtesy of Ricardo Ronderos, Universidad Nacional de La Plata, Argentina

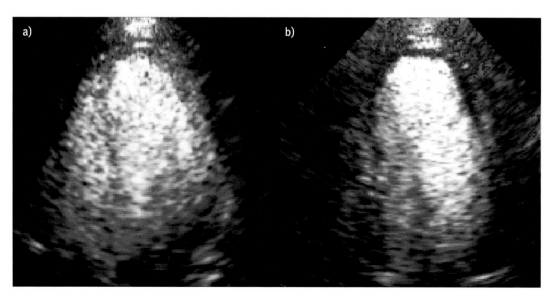

Fig. 30 Real-time resting myocardial contrast studies using power pulse inversion imaging following 0.3ml Optison. (a) Normal patient. (b) Patient with an extensive resting apical perfusion defect due to previous infarction. Power pulse inversion frame rates were 15Hz at an MI of 0.1–0.15.
Courtesy of Thomas Porter and Feng Xie, University of Nebraska, NE, USA

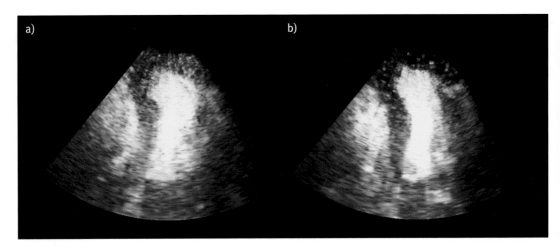

Fig. 31 Harmonic power Doppler, four chamber view, infusion of Levovist. Example of shorter pulsing interval revealing apical perfusion defect. A defect is hardly visualised at 5:1 pulsing interval (a), but clearly visible at 1:1 (b).

flow in perfusion beds distal to a significant coronary stenosis is not changed by stress, therefore longer intervals are needed to opacify the myocardium. With longer trigger intervals the hypoperfused volume of tissue still contains less microbubbles than the adjacent normally perfused areas. However, the differences in bubble concentration between normal and hypoperfused areas may not be sufficiently high to provide adequate visualisation of the perfusion deficit, which can therefore be overlooked. Real-time perfusion imaging of replenishment following one or several destruction frames, provides multiple frames with different concentrations of myocardial contrast. Therefore, the opportunity to create an optimal display of a perfusion defect should be higher than with triggered imaging. Clinical studies are in progress to investigate this hypothesis.

Evaluation of the perfusion defects is further complicated by effect of respiratory and scanhead movement on the signal intensities. Visual judgement should always be made using a series of frames rather than single ones. Because of the high number of frames needed for-side-by-side comparisons of rest and stress images, arrangement of digitally stored data on a computer is most convenient. Having the recordings on a computer further facilitates the use of advanced methods for quantitative analysis, which may complete the visual evaluation (see Chapter 4). Since conventional stress echo is often performed in conjunction with a perfusion study, acquisition analysis of MCE recordings is ideally implemented into the stress echo recording package on the scanner.

> **Calling a perfusion defect**
>
> A visually evident contrast defect is considered present when there is a relative decrease in contrast enhancement in one region compared with other adjacent regions, which have the same or worse imaging conditions.

3.9.2 Visual assessment of post-processed recordings

Post processing of myocardial perfusion images is necessary when harmonic B-mode or pulse inversion imaging is used (Figure 32). This is because of the small incremental enhancement provided by contrast over the background tissue harmonic echo. Several offline imaging analysis tools are available for this task, which requires digital recording of both baseline and contrast enhanced images. Before subtraction two tasks must be carried out. First, grey levels in the image, which are logarithmically mapped from the echo level received by the scanner, must be converted to a linear scale. If this is not done – for example if two images recorded on videotape are simply subtracted – the resulting image will depend on machine settings, attenuation and other factors unrelated to the amount of contrast in the myocardium, and essentially be meaningless. Second, the images must be aligned so that the subtracted quantities correspond to the same anatomic area. Because the heart has complex movement and because the baseline and contrast images are acquired at different times, this is not a trivial challenge. The process is described in detail in §4.2.2.

3.9.3 Reporting visual judgement

We have developed reporting forms for perfusion studies similar to those used in conventional stress echocardiography (Figure 33).

Criteria for visual assessment of MCE studies		
	Rest	**Stress**
Normal perfusion	Moderate or strong contrast enhancement (score 2 or 3) at least at higher trigger intervals (1:3 or 1:5) (contrast enhancement in basal segments may be poor)	Moderate or strong signals at low trigger interval (1:1) Increase of signal intensities at higher trigger intervals
Fixed perfusion defect (Subendocardial or transmural)	No or poor contrast enhancement (score 0 or 1)*	No or poor contrast enhancement (score 0 or 1)*
Reversible perfusion defect (subendocardial or transmural)	Moderate or adequate contrast enhancement (score 2 or 3) at least at higher trigger intervals (1:3 or 1:5)	Poor signals at low trigger interval (1:1)*

* Moderate or strong enhancement in adjacent segments with similar or worse imaging conditions

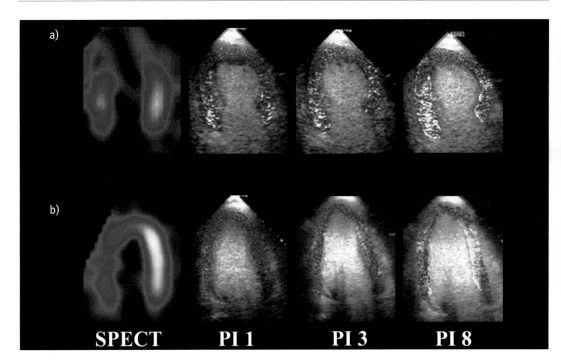

Fig. 32 B-mode harmonic recordings (four chamber view) after background subtraction and colour coding, comparison with SPECT. Effect of increasing pulsing intervals of an anteroapical (a) and inferoposterior (b) myocardial infarction.
Courtesy of Jonathan Lindner and Sanjiv Kaul, University of Virginia, Charlottesville, VI, USA

First, the segments in each scanplane are evaluated for contrast enhancement using the three step scoring as shown in §3.9.1. If a segment cannot be evaluated because of wall motion artifacts or attenuation, it is marked with an 'X'. This is repeated for the rest and stress images, which are then compared. To describe the changes between baseline and stress recordings, a judgement is made as to whether there is increased (+), decreased (-), no change (0) in contrast compared to baseline. If no signals are visible in a segment at both baseline and stress, this segment cannot be used for assessment of stress changes and is marked with an 'X'.

Visual judgement is summarised using the following statements:

1. Which segments can be evaluated? It is not always necessary to have the information for the entire myocardium. If, for instance, the study is performed to assess the hemodynamic relevance of an LAD stenosis, it is sufficient to see septal and anterior segments. In this case normal or abnormal findings only pertain to the LAD territory. This is different from myocardial scintigraphy, where perfusion is always evaluated in the entire myocardium.

2. Judgement as to whether those segments seen are normal or abnormal according to the criteria listed in the following Tables.

3. The results of the advanced methods for analysis of myocardial contrast studies may be

added to the report as soon there are reference values (see Chapter 4).

4. A brief indication as to which coronary artery is thought to be involved.

3.10 Interpretation of myocardial contrast echo: clinical profiles

3.10.1 Acute myocardial infarction

In acute transmural myocardial infarction there is a high grade or complete reduction of perfusion in a particular area of the myocardium. Therefore no, or only slight contrast will be found in this area following intravenous injection of the contrast agent (Figure 34). As long as there is complete occlusion of the epicardial vessel, the entire wall will show either no contrast signals or reduced filling if collateral blood flow is present. After restoration of blood flow, contrast will fill in those areas with preserved microvascular integrity, which is a prerequisite for myocardial viability (Figure 35). Thus areas with complete necrosis will show no refilling with contrast after successful reopening of the occluded coronary artery. Preliminary clinical studies have demonstrated the usefulness of contrast echo in the evaluation of patients with acute myocardial infarction (14, 15, 17, 36–42). Figure 36 shows a

When is a perfusion defect real?	
Criteria for a real perfusion defect (four chamber view)	
Decrease of contrast enhancement in:	**compared to:**
Apical septum	Mid and basal septum, lateral wall
Mid septum	Mid and basal lateral wall
Basal septum	Basal lateral wall
Apical lateral wall	Mid and basal lateral wall
Mid lateral wall	Basal lateral wall
Basal lateral wall	Not available
Criteria for a real perfusion defect (two chamber view)	
Decrease of contrast enhancement in:	**compared to:**
Apical inferior wall	Mid and basal inferior wall, anterior wall
Mid inferior wall	Mid and basal anterior wall
Basal inferior wall	Basal anterior wall
Apical anterior wall	Mid and basal inferior wall
Mid anterior wall	Basal inferior wall
Basal anterior wall	Not available

Rheinische Friedrich-Wilhelms-Universität

Medizinische Klinik und Poliklinik II
Innere Medizin —Kardiologie — Pneumologie
Direktor: Prof. Dr. B. Lüderitz

Medizinische Einrichtungen
Sigmund-Freud-Str. 25
53105 Bonn

CONTRAST ECHOCARDIOGRAPHY

name: _____
ward: _____
date: _____
study enrollment? _____

TTE rest ☐
TTE stress ☐

Adenosine ○
Dipyridamol ○
Dobutamine ○

Myocardial Contrast Enhancement

REST	STRESS	COMPARISON: REST/ STRESS

Score:
0 = no contrast enhancement
1 = poor/ incomplete contrast enhancement
2 = moderate contrast enhancement
3 = strong/ complete contrast enhancement
X = not available (wall motion artefacts, attenuation, contrast shadowing)

Score:
0 = no change
+ = increased myocardial contrast compared to baseline
− = decreased myocardial contrast compared to baseline
X = not available

EVALUATION:

Fig. 33 Report form for visual assessment of a myocardial perfusion study.

flow chart for the use of contrast echo in the setting of acute myocardial infarction. Although only preliminary clinical studies are available, the lack of effective alternatives for assessment of reperfusion may be sufficient justification for using contrast echo if the guidelines for exclusion of false defects are taken into account.

3.10.2 Scar or fibrosis versus viable myocardium

Necrotic tissue and the evolving scar are displayed as fixed defects. They have no or minimal rest perfusion, because the microvascular network has been damaged irreversibly during ischemia (Figures 37, 38, 39). In contrast, viable myocardium – stunned or hibernating – still has its microvascular network, which can be imaged

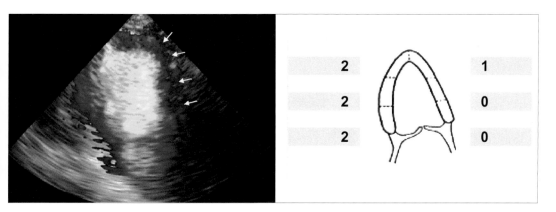

Fig. 34 Harmonic power Doppler (apical two chamber view, Levovist infusion). Apical and anterior wall perfusion defect (arrows) shown in anterolateral myocardial infarction.
Courtesy of Folkert Ten Cate, Thoraxcenter, Rotterdam, Netherlands

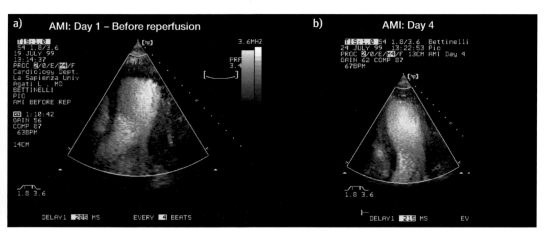

Fig. 35 Harmonic Power Doppler, four chamber view, Levovist infusion. Large apical defect in acute apicoseptal infarction (a) and after successful reperfusion (b).
Courtesy of Luciano Agati, University of Rome, Italy

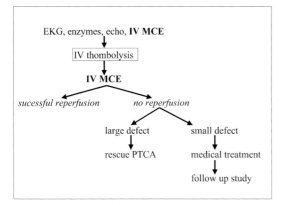

Fig. 36 Use of myocardial contrast echo in the management of acute transmural myocardial infarction.

using contrast echo. It should be remembered that contrast echo provides information on microvascular integrity, not myocyte function. Absence of signal in an infarcted area represents no reflow or a fibrotic scar in the chronic phase. Whether the presence of contrast in the myocardium is an indicator of viability remains to be established. Studies using intra-arterial injections of contrast do suggest that the presence of signal in areas of damaged myocardium indicates viability (15), but little data are available for intravenous contrast imaging. Until trials establish ranges, evaluation of viability should be confined to differentiating between a definite lack of contrast and a strong and convincing contrast effect. Studies may be used in combination with other methods such as low dose dobutamine stress or positron emission tomography (PET).

It has been shown that the appearance of contrast and full filling may often be delayed markedly because the area of interest is supplied mainly by collaterals. Thus quantitative analysis should include longer trigger intervals (e.g. 1:10) to detect late filling.

3.10.3 Coronary artery stenosis

Perfusion defects during exercise, but normal perfusion at rest are the typical findings in the visual assessment of significant coronary stenoses (see §3.9.1.2). Figures 40–43 show examples with different imaging methods. Only with very severe stenosis is resting blood flow reduced and the defect visible at rest. In moderate epicardial stenosis (50–85 percent), myocardial blood flow is maintained at rest because the post-stenotic arterioles dilate. During exercise or pharmacological stress perfusion defects can be displayed because the ability to increase blood flow is reduced in regions supplied by coronary arteries with significant stenosis.

Reduction of myocardial blood flow is associated with a reduction of myocardial blood volume. Since ultrasound contrast agents are

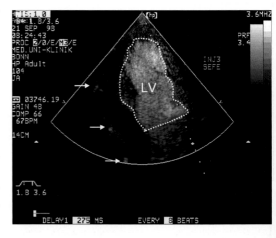

Fig. 37 Extended inferior infarction due to no reflow following reopening of the right coronary artery, two chamber view, harmonic power Doppler. Dotted line represents endocardial border. Note the absence of signals in the papillary muscle and entire inferior wall, compared to the signals in the anterior wall. There are only a few small epicardial vessels displayed on the inferior wall (arrows).

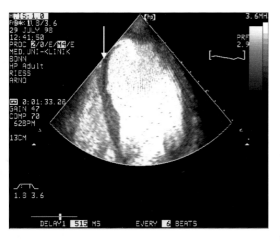

Fig. 38 Apicoseptal scar following myocardial infarction (harmonic power Doppler, four chamber view, Levovist infusion). Decreased signals in a thin subendocardial layer (arrow) compared to subepicardial layers.

pure intravascular tracers, the myocardial contrast signals have been used as an estimate of myocardial blood volume. The prerequisite for using contrast signals as an estimate of local blood volume is that the concentration of microbubbles in the blood is not different in the areas which are compared. This is true with a non-destructive imaging mode such as PPI. With a destructive bubble imaging technique like HPD myocardial contrast strength represents myocardial blood volume only if long trigger intervals are used (>1:5, see Chapter 4).

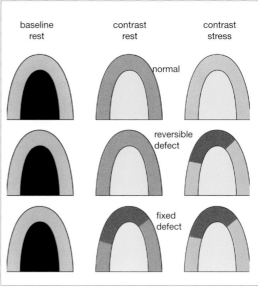

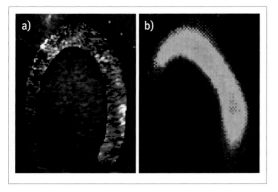

Fig. 39 Myocardial perfusion imaging at rest in a patient with remote inferior myocardial infarction. Left panel shows venous myocardial contrast echocardiography, harmonic B-mode, Levovist infusion, pulsing rate 1:7, background subtraction and colour coding. In the two chamber view a contrast defect of the inferior wall is visible. Corresponding vertical long axis on MIBI SPECT (b) shows missing tracer uptake in the same region.
Courtesy of Christian Firschke, Deutsches Herzzentrum, Technische Universität München, Germany

Fig. 40 Schematic changes in fixed and reversible perfusion defects in a two chamber view. Relative reduction of signal intensities is seen in the apical myocardium compared to the neighbouring segments at rest and during stress in a fixed defect, whereas the reversible defect is displayed only during stress. Note the increase in myocardial opacification observed during stress in normal myocardium.

With shorter trigger intervals the speed of replenishment of the disrupted microbubbles heavily determines myocardial contrast signal strength. During stress flow rate is increased in

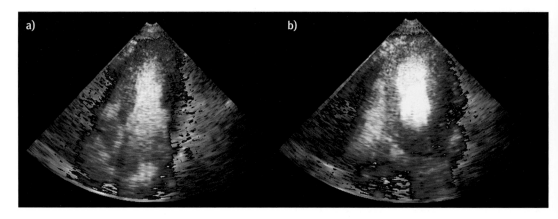

Fig. 41 Normal response to adenosine stress (harmonic power Doppler, four chamber view). Note increase in myocardial signal intensities in the adenosine recording (b) over the baseline image (a).

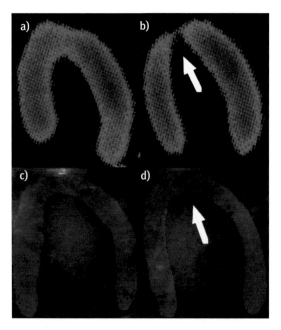

Fig. 42 Myocardial perfusion imaging at rest and with stress in a patient with a 58 percent diameter stenosis of mid LAD (segment 8) considered of uncertain functional relevance. Small reversible tracer uptake defect of the apical myocardium (arrow) on TC99m Sestamibi SPECT: horizontal long axis at rest (a) and with exercise (b). Corresponding homogeneous myocardial contrast during intraveous infusion of Levovist in the four chamber view at rest (c) and small contrast defect (arrow) during infusion of adenosine (d).
Courtesy of Christian Firschke, Deutsches Herzzentrum, Technische Universität München, Germany

regions supplied by normal epicardial coronary arteries and disrupted microbubbles are replenished during shorter time intervals than at rest. This is not possible in areas supplied by coronary arteries with significant stenosis.

Thus, at short trigger intervals myocardial contrast reflects flow, and is reduced in ischemic segments compared to areas supplied by normal coronary arteries.

Perfusion Imaging

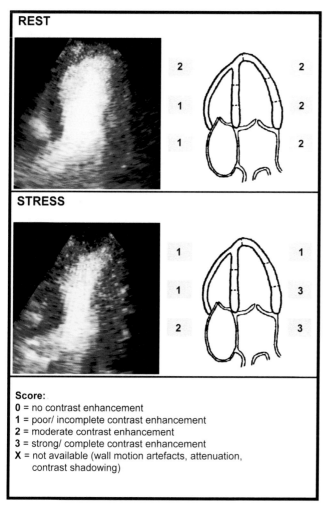
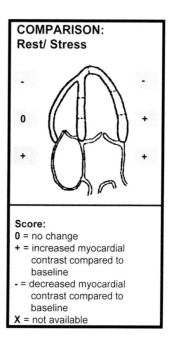

Fig. 43 Visual judgement of rest and adenosine stress images (harmonic power Doppler, four chamber view, trigger 1:3) in a patient with exertional chest pain using the report form presented in Fig. 29. Reduction of apical contrast signal intensity and no increase in septal signal strength compared to marked enhancement in the lateral wall. Corresponding findings in a Sestamibi SPECT, coronary angiography revealed 90 percent proximal LAD stenosis.

3.11 Pitfalls and troubleshooting

3.11.1 Inadequate myocardial contrast

Weak or absent myocardial contrast does not always mean impaired myocardial perfusion, but may be caused by technical problems. For reliable evaluation of perfusion, a minimum quantity of microbubbles need to be present in the myocardial vessels. However, complete absence of myocardial contrast despite cavity enhancement is often caused by inappropriate machine settings. Inadequate contrast dose should be considered after scanplane and instrument controls have been re-checked (see Table). Strong myocardial and cavity contrast signals in the nearfield but inadequate signals at greater depth are often caused by attenuation by the agent, which can be obviated by reducing the rate of agent infusion. In some instances, however, focus position in the nearfield can result in a similar contrast image.

Pitfalls in myocardial contrast echocardiography

- Inadequate myocardial contrast
- Contrast shadowing
- Blooming
- Wall motion artifacts

Weak or absent myocardial contrast after an initially adequate display may also be due to displacement of the scanhead. Triggered imaging is a challenge for both the investigator and the patient. Dyspnea during vasodilator stress and atypical chest pain cause deep breaths and loss of the imaging plane. In this situation it is necessary to leave the triggered mode and to use continuous scanning to readjust the scanplane (with harmonic power Doppler, harmonic B-mode should be used for optimising the scanplane). Beware that at high MI, this process depletes the systemic level of the agent during the infusion, to the extent that one must wait for about two minutes for the contrast level to recover before starting to scan again. After readjustment of the scanplane, triggered imaging can be initiated to complete the protocol, discarding the first frame.

Appparent defects in the lateral wall often do not represent a real perfusion deficit, but inadequate myocardial contrast. Similarly, false-positive defects may be found in the anterior wall. Extracardiac attenuation by ribs and pulmonary tissue may be the reasons for lower amounts of acoustic power being delivered to the lateral wall in the four chamber view and the anterior wall in the two chamber view. Sometimes this is so severe that complete shadowing of the deeper-lying structures occurs. Shadowing is recognised by the abrupt weakening of echoes distal to a point in the scan line. This shadowing line is often found laterally of the endocardial border and so is sometimes only identifiable with the contrast

Troubleshooting for inadequate myocardial contrast

Weak/absent contrast in the entire myocardium
1. Check scanplane in harmonic B-mode
2. Check machine settings
3. Check venous line, stopcock
4. Check infusion pump: running, correct setting
   If all are set correctly, increase infusion speed

Weak/absent myocardial contrast at greater depth but strong signals in the nearfield
1. Check whether focus position is correct
2. Check for contrast shadowing, reduce infusion speed if necessary

Weak/absent myocardial contrast after initial adequate display
Displacement of the scanhead
Readjust during continuous harmonic B-mode
Check for systemic depletion of bubbles following real-time imaging

Weak/absent myocardial contrast in the lateral sectors of the imaging field
1. Rule out extra-cardiac shadowing (ribs, pulmonary tissue)
2. Check myocardial grey level in harmonic B-mode
3. Adjust scanplane to show lateral structures in centre of sector
4. Exclude attenuation by cavity contrast (reduced intensity of cavity signals close to the lateral wall)

agent. If shadowing is detected, the scanplane should be modified using continuous harmonic B-mode so that the lateral wall is centred in the imaging field. The aim is for the lateral and anterior walls to be displayed with grey myocardium. However, difficulty with the lateral wall is common even when these measures have been taken. An apparent isolated defect in the lateral wall should therefore always be treated with caution.

3.11.2 Contrast shadowing

Weak or absent myocardial contrast at greater depth when there are strong signals in the nearfield is probably caused by cavity bubbles shadowing distal regions (Figures 44, 45). Shadowing by the contrast agent is a particular problem for myocardial contrast echo, because higher concentrations of bubbles are needed. Those present in the nearfield attenuate the sound to the point that bubble disruption does not occur at greater depth. Thus the basal septum (four chamber view), basal inferior wall (two chamber view) and particularly basal lateral wall (four chamber view) can have 'pseudo' defects in healthy subjects. The problem is more serious for parasternal than for apical views, because the ultrasound must penetrate both the RV and LV cavities to reach the inferior or posterior LV wall. The RV may attenuate more, because it contains larger bubbles wich have not been filtered by the lungs. So far there is no way to compensate for attenuation, but there are some guidelines for its reduction.

Most important is to use the lowest effective dose of contrast. Particularly for quantitative analysis, it is an advantage not to have a bright myocardium with large quantities of microbubbles. When the patient is scheduled for a stress study a dramatic increase in signal intensity must be anticipated. The protocols provided in the tables on pages 103, 104 and 107, 108 aim for the highest sensitivity with the lowest doses of contrast. Since the optimal dose for the individual cannot be predicted, it should be determined empirically, and adjustment of a contrast infusion is the best way to do this. Note that changes in infusion rate take up to two minutes to become effective, so

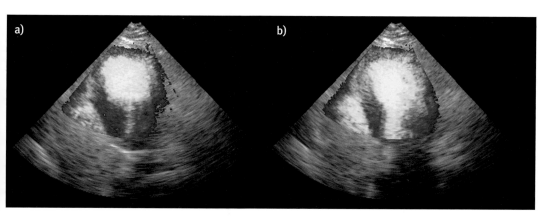

Fig. 44 Contrast shadowing due overdosing of contrast (a). With no power Doppler signals at greater depth, better penetration after reduction of infusion rate (b).

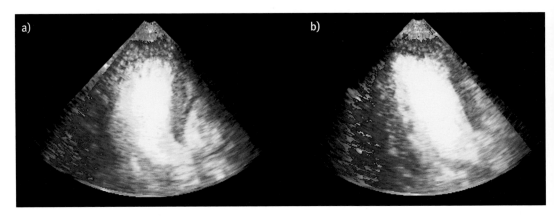

Fig. 45 False defect due to attenuation in the basal posterolateral wall using harmonic power Doppler mode (long axis view). (a) Defect using standard scanplane. After changing transducer position with posterolateral wall located closer to the centre of the sector, the false defect disappeared (b).

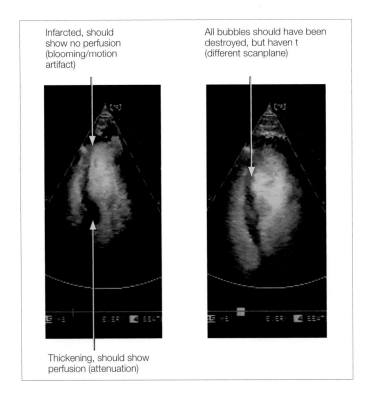

Fig. 46 Perfusion imaging artifacts: 63-year-old man with recent anterior MI and mid LAD occlusion, double frame triggered harmonic power Doppler, four chamber view. Notice the different scanplane with a larger LV cavity in frame two compared to frame one. Although consecutive frames are acquired, there has been considerable cardiac movement in between due to the low frame rate of harmonic power Doppler. The basal septal defect is caused by attenuation, the infarcted area is hardly visualised because of blooming or wall motion artifacts.
Courtesy of Jim Thomas, Cleveland Clinic, OH, USA

should be avoided during data acquisition. The contrast dose is better adjusted before starting the acquisition protocol. However, the dramatic increase in signal intensity following vasodilator administration may cause attenuation problems despite optimal recordings at rest. In this situation it is better to complete the protocol and repeat the acquisition of the vasodilator images at a lower infusion rate. The comparison of rest and stress studies performed with different doses of contrast is permissible, when relative measurements are used instead of absolute intensity measurements.

3.11.3 Blooming

Blooming describes the appearance of contrast signals which originate from the myocardial tissue but spread into neighbouring compartments. This phenomenon occurs when cavity signals are strong and is found both in harmonic power Doppler and greyscale techniques (harmonic B-mode and pulse inversion). There are two types of blooming: with cavity blooming, the cavity signals exceed the endocardial borders to a certain extent and resemble myocardial opacification (Figure 46). As intense opacification of the cavities of the heart is always detectable with intravenous administration of contrast agent, blooming must be expected. Sceptics of myocardial contrast echocardiography maintain that the myocardial signals are largely due to blooming after intravenous administration of contrast agent. However, this speculation is easily dismissed. Following an IV bolus, there is a clear delay between the appearance of signal in the left ventricle and its appearance in the myocardium. Furthermore, the more macular and reticular distribution pattern – corresponding to the intramyocardial vessels – at low trigger rates cannot be accounted for by blooming artifacts. With blooming alone, a homogeneous contrast effect would be expected in the subendocardial layers. While blooming does occur, it can be distinguished from real perfusion.

Cavity blooming is caused by strong echoes which lie above or below the scan plane. Strong echoes can particularly be formed in the septum from blooming of the right-ventricular cavity. Such septal blooming then occurs simultaneously with the maximum contrast effect in the right ventricle, clearly before the time at which myocardial perfusion is displayed. This phenomenon can be seen during bolus injections. With a proper rate of contrast agent infusion, cavity blooming is less common. The immediate subendocardial area of 1 mm should be omitted if a region of interest is sited for quantitative analysis in the myocardium.

Blooming of the intramyocardial vessels also occurs (48). The vessels displayed in the ultrasound image appear much wider than in reality (Figure 47). This is mainly due to the physical and technical limitations of ultrasound equipment, whose resolution is currently 1–2 mm. Most intramyocardial vessels have a considerably smaller diameter so that an exact representation is not possible. Blooming of intramyocardial vessels may be of benefit for visual assessment because the very small vessels are appreciated more easily. They may, however, bias quantitative assessment if the region-of-interest is too small and contains such a vessel.

3.11.4 Wall motion artifacts

Motion artifacts are most important in harmonic power Doppler. Wall motion artifacts

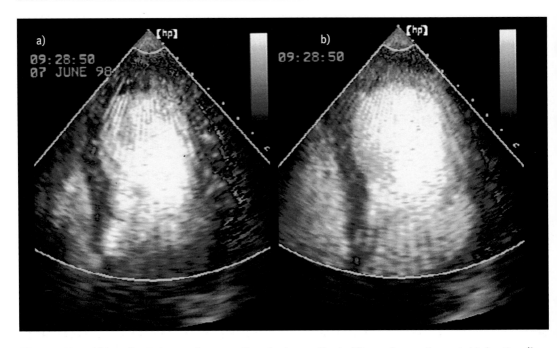

Fig. 47 Vessel blooming in harmonic power Doppler in a patient with previous apicoseptal infarction (four chamber view). (a) shows recording at a trigger rate of 1:1 with display of blooming intramyocardial vessels – particularly in the lateral wall. (b) A homogenous myocardial contrast pattern is found in the lateral wall using 1:4 trigger rate due to additional filling of small intramyocardial vessels. Notice the reduced contrast in the septum compared to the lateral wall.

have already been mentioned in §3.6.1.1 as a pitfall during contrast enhanced power Doppler for LV opacification, where they usually do not have a great impact on endocardial border delineation. During assessment of myocardial perfusion, wall motion artifacts can distort the display of myocardial contrast. They can mimic tissue perfusion signals if they are not eliminated by the pre-contrast settings. However, even after successful suppression of wall motion artifacts at baseline some may be encountered during contrast enhancement. These may be due to unexpected respiratory or thoracic movement and occur with the contrast signals from intramyocardial vessels. Such artifacts are often confined to a few frames, which should be excluded from further processing.

Using short trigger intervals only the larger vessels are filled with contrast. Their characteristic pattern is easy to distinguish from wall motion artifact, which often is not confined to myocardial tissue (Figure 48). At longer trigger intervals, perfusion contrast becomes more homogeneous and recognition of wall motion artifacts more difficult. They can be recognised as flash-like coloured areas (changing from frame to frame) which often overlay epi- or pericardial layers of the lateral wall (four chamber view), but may be found in other regions such as near the mitral valve and the septum. Structures with high backscatter and fast movement parallel to the beam are prone to produce motion artifacts, which are often therefore found in fibrotic pericardial layers and perivalvular tissue.

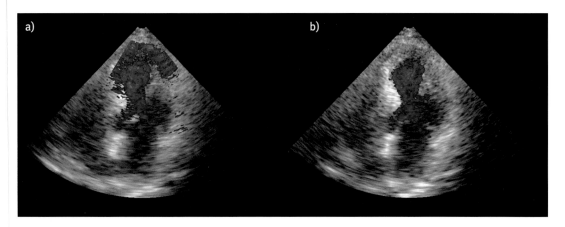

Fig. 48 Apical wall motion artifacts to respiratory motion (a), complete disappearance during shallow respiration (b).

In single contrast enhanced frames it may be difficult to distinguish between wall motion artifact and perfusion signals. Here, reviewing consecutive frames acquired with the same trigger intervals is very helpful: any abrupt change in signal pattern should make one think of a wall motion artifact. It is always necessary to review a series of frames (for example, five) taken at the same machine setting during infusion of the agent.

3.11.5 The bubble depletion artifact

The intention of an infusion is to maintain a steady level of enhancement in the myocardium. However, the imaging frame used to destroy the agent in the myocardium also destroys agent in the cavities. As more destruction frames are used at shorter trigger intervals, the systemic pool of the agent begins to become depleted and its concentration drop. Shorter trigger intervals have the ability to reduce the systemic level of contrast to the extent that the myocardial signal is lowered artifactually. In some cases, this can result in an incorrect reperfusion curve and a misinterpretation of the images. Inadvertant bubble depletion can also occur after a period of high MI continuous imaging (for example to adjust the scanplane during a triggered study). Power pulse inversion, which uses an MI so low that the agent is not destroyed as it is imaged, is not susceptible to this artifact.

Coronary Flow Reserve*

3.12 Coronary flow reserve and myocardial contrast echo

Measurement of coronary flow reserve is a procedure to assess myocardial ischemia in a quantitative way. Since coronary flow and tissue perfusion are linked, changes in myocardial tissue perfusion following a vasodilator stimulus should provide complemetary information. However, myocardial contrast echo has the same limitations as SPECT in detecting balanced hypoperfusion in, for example, three-

*This section courtesy of Carlo Caiati, University of Cagliari, Italy

Clinical methods to assess CFR		
Methodology	**Pros**	**Cons**
Positron emission tomography (PET)	Non-invasive, global and regional myocardial perfusion reserve objectively assessable	Scarce Radiation exposure Expensive
Intracoronary Doppler flow wire	Precise post-stenotic CFR assessment Evaluation of relative and fractional coronary flow reserve Difficult to repeat	Invasive and risky Expensive
Transesophageal Doppler echocardiography (TEE)	Widely available	Semi-invasive Limited prediction of coronary stenosis Limited to LAD
Transthoracic contrast Doppler echocardiography	Non invasive, widely available Optimal prediction of coronary stenosis Technically feasible with harmonic contrast imaging	Limited to LAD

approximately 10–20 percent of patients with exercise-induced coronary insufficiency. An abnormal CFR finding confirms the cardiac origin of the chest pain and rules out false positive stress testing. CFR can be impaired by a variety of disorders of the microcirculation. Pharmacologic interventions of these disorders can be easily assessed by CFR measurement. Diabetes, arterial hypertension or hypercholesteremia, for example, are associated with impaired CFR (61–63).

3.14.1 Selection of patients

A suboptimal ultrasound window, a major concern in any ultrasound approach, does not reduce the feasibility of CFR measurements if the combination of second harmonic imaging and a contrast agent is used. In our experience the feasibility of almost 100 percent has been confirmed in large series of patients including those with large body habitus (59, 62).

Contrast enhancement should always be used even when good Doppler quality is achieved at baseline without enhancement. Contrast helps maintain good monitoring of the Doppler signal from the LAD during hyperemia, where vasodilators induced hyperpnea and tachycardia make an adequate blood flow Doppler recording more difficult. In cases with good signal at baseline a very small amount of contrast can be used just for the hyperemic portion of the study.

> **Indications for transthoracic Doppler of LAD flow**
>
> - Before coronary angiography
>   Suspected LAD stenosis (previous anterior infarction, stress ECG, stress echo, myocardial scintigraphy)
>   Myocardial contrast echo
>
> - After coronary angiography – LAD stenosis
>   Significance of stenosis
>   (in combination with myocardial contrast)
>
> - After coronary angiography – normal coronary arteries
>   To confirm cardiac origin of chest pain
>   To control therapeutic interventions

3.15 How to perform a CFR study

3.15.1 Intravenous lines

Two intravenous lines are needed for studies using adenosine as vasodilator. An indwelling cannula (20 gauge or less) is inserted into a cubital vein for the infusion of the contrast agent. Another line is necessary for infusion of adenosine, this line can have a smaller size (22 gauge). Interactions between adenosine and contrast agents are unlikely, but have not been systematically evaluated so far. Thus infusing adenosine and contrast agent via the same line cannot be recommended. If dipyridamole is used for induction of hyperemia, only one venous line is needed, because the vasodilator effect persists after dipyridamole has been infused and simultaneous infusion with the echo contrast agent is not necessary.

3.15.2 Contrast agent

All available contrast agents can be used to enhance Doppler signals. Infusion of the contrast agent is necessary to maintain the same level of contrast enhancement during baseline and hyperemia. This method of administration has the advantage of maintaining enhancement over several minutes, without affecting the peak intensity that is attained. In comparison to myocardial contrast echo, doses of echo contrast are much lower. An example of a dose regimen for Levovist is: one vial prepared using a concentration of 300 mg/ml. The agent is administered by infusion using an infusion pump connected over a special 50-cm connector tubing. The initial infusion rate is 1 ml/min. This rate can be increased to a maximum of 2 ml/min or decreased to a minimum of 0.5 ml/min, according to the quality of the Doppler signal obtained.

> **CFR in the 'difficult' echo patient**
>
> CFR measurements can be performed in patients with poor windows where myocardial contrast echocardiography is not recommended

3.15.3 Protocols to induce hyperemia

The dipyridamole and adenosine protocols which are established for regular stress echo and SPECT are useful for assessment of CFR too (see Figures 49, 50). For dipyridamole, only one venous line is necessary but more contrast agent is needed: because of the delay between the start of the drug and achieving complete vasodilatatory effect (6–8 minutes for the low dose and 12–14 min for the high dose), two separate contrast infusions need to be given. This also implies that LAD flow needs to be re-imaged during dipyridamole as the spot is usually lost at the end of the contrast enhancement for the baseline acquisition.

Steps to perform a CFR study

1. Insert an indwelling cannula (20 gauge) into a cubital vein. Connect the line for contrast infusion
2. Insert an indwelling cannula (22 gauge or more) into a forearm vein (only for adenosine). Connect the line with adenosine infusion
3. Prepare contrast agent and adenosine infusion
4. Search for LAD flow using fundamental colour Doppler
5. Start contrast infusion
6. Search for LAD flow using harmonic colour Doppler
7. Switch to fundamental (harmonic) PW Doppler, record LAD flow at rest
8. Start adenosine infusion
9. Record LAD flow during hyperemia

Intravenous adenosine (140 µg/kg/min over 6 minutes) seems superior to dipyridamole. First, adenosine acts rapidly, achieving peak effect in about 55 seconds compared to about 100 seconds with dipyridamole (64). This shortens the hyperemic part of the study to 2–3 minutes so that a single contrast infusion of 11 ml volume is sufficient for all of the examination. Second, because the enhancement of the Doppler signal is obtained without interruption, the Doppler recording is more easily and accurately performed. Third, unlike dipyridamole, adenosine in doses >100 µg/kg has been shown to be nearly equivalent to papaverine to produce maximal coronary vaso-

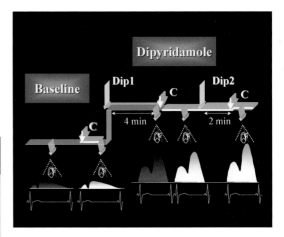

Fig. 49 Protocol for dipyridamole stress, DIP1 = 0.56 mg/kg over 4 minutes, DIP2 = 0.28 mg/kg over 2 minutes

dilation. Fourth, the short duration of the examination combined with the prompt reversibility of the side effects, if any, after termination of the infusion make this drug safe and acceptable to the patient. The only shortcomings of adenosine are 1) the need of two intravenous lines, 2) the higher cost, and 3) the frequently induced hyperpnea. Hyperpnea, however, may be disturbing for the patient, but rarely causes degradation of image quality.

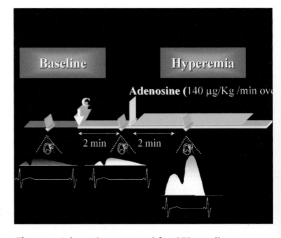

Fig. 50 Adenosine protocol for CFR studies

3.15.4 Image orientation for visualising blood flow in the LAD

A systematic attempt must be made to record flow in the distal or in the mid part of the LAD (Figure 51). The approach for the distal part consists first in obtaining a short axis of the left ventricular apex and of the anterior groove. Thereafter, a search for coronary flow in the anterior groove is started. When a diastolic flow, circularly-shaped vessel is recognised in the anterior groove area, it is brought into the central part of the ultrasound field by angling laterally and slightly above the central ray of the scan plane. At this point, the transducer should be rotated counterclockwise to obtain the best long axis colour view. Alternatively, in order to achieve a better alignment between flow and the ultrasound beam, a modified foreshortened two chamber view can be obtained by sliding the transducer superiorly and medially from an apical two chamber position. In this way visualisation of the epicardial part of the anterior wall is obtained with less pulmonary interference. The mid part of the LAD is visualised by a low parasternal short axis view of the base of the heart modified by a slight clockwise rotation of the beam in order to bring into view the anterior groove area and thereby the mid portion of the LAD that runs over the left border of the right ventricular outflow tract (post-pulmonary tract). Pulsed wave flow Doppler recording in the LAD is first attempted at baseline in fundamental mode, and after contrast in harmonic mode.

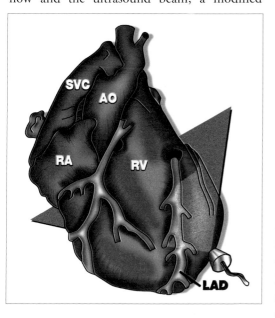

Fig. 51 Plane orientation for acquisition of LAD flow: the mid part of the LAD is visualised by a low parasternal short axis view of the base of the heart modified by a slight clockwise rotation of the beam in order to bring into view the anterior groove area.

3.15.5 Instrument settings

All the setting adjustments described here have been established using the Acuson Sequoia system. First, regular tissue harmonic mode with the default settings is used to obtain a short axis of the left ventricular apex and of the anterior groove. Then fundamental colour Doppler is used to search the LAD. As soon as LAD flow has been identified, the contrast infusion is started and harmonic colour Doppler mode initialised. The harmonic colour Doppler setting should be adjusted to maximise scanning sensitivity without reducing the frame rate. The pulse repetition frequency is decreased by changing the colour Doppler velocity scale (between 11 and 25 cm/s), gate size should be maximally increased, gain increased until noise begins to appear faintly and colour Doppler box size kept small. Colour transmit power is turned up to the maximum level. Increasing ultrasound energy to maximum level (destruction mode) is important during contrast administration in

B-mode and colour Doppler for CFR: settings

B-Mode:

Transducer	Normal
Scanning modality	Tissue harmonic
Transmit power	Maximum (0 dB), as optimised for tissue harmonics
General gain	Default (0 dB)
TGC	Keep low; (high B-mode gain hampers colour flow display)
Depth	Reduce depth (to increase frame rate)

Colour Doppler before contrast:

Transducer	Normal
Scanning modality	Fundamental velocity colour Doppler (2.5 MHz)
Transmit Power	Maximum (0 dB)
Sample volume size	Maximum (3) (to increase sensitivity)
Gain	Set high, at the level at which noise begins to appear faintly
Colour Doppler box size	Keep as small as possible (to increase frame rate)
Pulse repetition frequency (PRF)	Decrease to improve sensitivity (velocity range 14-18 cm/s)

Colour Doppler after contrast:

Transducer	Normal
Scanning modality	Harmonic colour Doppler (1.7 MHz transmit/3.5 MHz receive)
Transmit Power	Maximum (0 dB) (destruction mode)
Gain	Unchanged or slightly reduced
Colour Doppler box size	Unchanged
Pulse repetition frequency (PRF)	Unchanged or a little increased (to reduce flash artifacts caused by the increased heart rate)

order to maximise harmonic production by the microbubbles and so for optimising coronary flow recording with harmonic colour Doppler.

With fundamental spectral Doppler, gain and transmit power are slightly reduced (-4 and -7 dB respectively) in order to avoid excessive spectral blooming during contrast administration. During contrast administration this setting does not generally need to be modified except on some occasions where, during spectral recording transmit power needs to be lowered a little in order to reduce disturbing vertical spikes caused by ultrasound breaking

Spectral Doppler for CFR: settings

Spectral Doppler before contrast:

Transducer	2–3 MHz sector
Scanning modality	Fundamental (2.5 MHz)
Sample volume size	4 mm
Transmit power	From –4 to –7 dB
Gain	From –4 to –7 dB
Dynamic range	Default (50 dB)

Spectral Doppler after contrast:

Transducer	2–3 MHz sector
Scanning modality	Fundamental (2.5 MHz)
Sample volume size	4 mm
Transmit Power	Unchanged or slightly reduced (to reduce "bubble noise")
Gain	Unchanged or a slightly reduced (to reduce blooming)
Dynamic range	Default (50 dB)

bubbles, the so called 'bubble noise' phenomenon (see §3.17.4). To measure coronary flow, colour flow imaging is used as a guide. Sample volume is positioned at the location of the vessel. Because of the absence of ventricular contraction in diastole, the position of the left anterior descending coronary artery is more stable in this part of the cardiac cycle, thus facilitating sample volume positioning.

3.15.6 Combination with myocardial contrast echo (MCE)

CFR measurements may be made in conjunction with myocardial contrast echocardiography. For this purpose the MCE study has to be performed with an adenosine infusion. After the MCE protocol has been completed, the adenosine infusion and contrast infusion are maintained and LAD flow is recorded. Usually transmit power needs to be reduced to avoid blooming and saturation of the LAD flow signals. Afterwards adenosine infusion is stopped but the contrast infusion continued and 20 seconds later the baseline LAD flow is recorded. This procedure can be performed within one minute, if the right plane for interrogating the LAD is quickly found. With some practice the sonographer will be able to easily find the LAD, because the colour and PW signals are very strong during contrast enhancement. The time to search for the LAD can further be reduced if the sonographer has identified the imaging plane during the baseline study.

3.16 Image acquisition and interpretation

Once adequate Doppler spectra are visible, recordings are started. It is useful to store a short period in colour mode with the cursor and sample volume in the LAD, to establish the Doppler angle, which must remain constant. For PW Doppler, at least five frames should be stored on videotape and/or cineloop. Recording of hyperemic flow velocity by PW Doppler is started as soon as the colour signal shows an increase in velocity, or in any case, within two minutes of the beginning of the adenosine infusion. It is continued until the 5th minute. If the Doppler angle or LAD segment appears different during the infusion to that seen at baseline, a new baseline velocity recording must be made. This can be done five minutes after the end of the infusion. It is best to maintain monitoring throughout the wash-out phase.

The recordings are analysed offline using the tools available in every Doppler system (Figure 52). Velocity-time integrals (VTI) are obtained by tracing the envelope of the Doppler spectra.

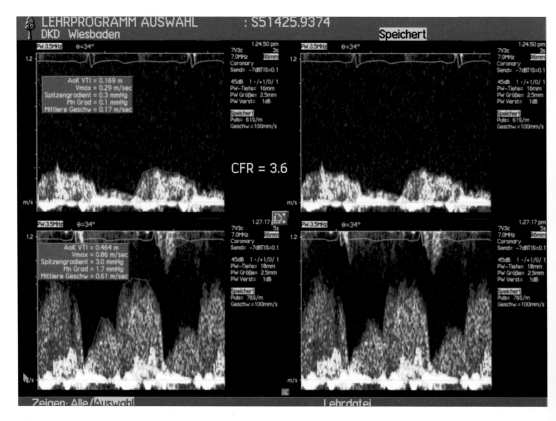

Fig. 52 Contrast enhanced pulsed wave Doppler tracings of LAD flow at rest (top) and during adenosine infusion (bottom). CFR is assessed by tracing the envelope of the Doppler spectra and calculating the velocity-time integrals. The ratio of adenosine to baseline data represents CFR.
Courtesy of Heinz Lambertz, Deutsche Klinik für Diagnostik Wiesbaden, Germany

An average of at least 3 cardiac cycles is made. The ratio of VTI during hyperemia to the VTI at baseline is the coronary flow reserve. If a CFR > 2.0 is considered normal and CFR < 2.0 abnormal, the sensitivity and specificity for detecting a >75 percent diameter LAD stenosis is 91 and 76 percent respectively.

3.16.1 Significance of an LAD stenosis

Coronary angiography provides little insight into the physiological significance of coronary stenoses, especially those of intermediate severity (65). Understanding functional impact of a stenosis is important for clinical decision making, as PTCA can be deferred safely in patients with intermediate stenosis but an adequate CFR value (66) as shown on Figure 53.

Coronary angiography (Figure 53 a) showed an apparently significant stenosis in the mid-LAD. In order to confirm its functional significance, a TTE CFR was performed (Figure 53 b) which showed a normal CFR. This was in agreement with adenosine/baseline 99 mTc-Sestamibi SPECT that did not show any reversible perfusion defect.

3.16.2 Follow-up of an LAD stenosis after PTCA

After PTCA, CFR recovers dramatically, reaching the lower limit of the normal range. The baseline diastolic/systolic ratio also returns to normal. The normalisation of diastolic/systolic ratio after PTCA could be a more specific index for successful recanalisation than CFR since CFR can still be depressed immediately after intervention (so-called 'microcirculation stunning') (67). Figure 54 is a typical example. Before PTCA the CFR was flat; in addition the ratio of the diastolic to systolic velocity is 1 (which is abnormal). After PTCA the ratio increased.

3.17 Pitfalls and troubleshooting

3.17.1 Angle of the vessel to the beam

One of the basic assumptions of the method is that the Doppler angle is kept constant throughout the examination. One way to reach this goal is to maintain the same view throughout the examination with no interruption of imaging. In this respect the use of adenosine protocol has eased the method enormously. However, in some cases there can still be some uncertainty. It is a good idea to check the constancy of the Doppler angle by verifying that the depth of the sample volume is the same throughout the examination. This only makes sense if the tomographic plane does not

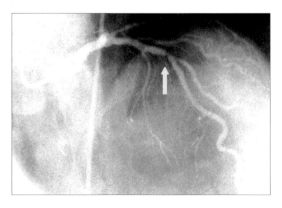

Fig. 53a Coronary angiogram in a patient with prolonged chest pain: 60 percent stenois in the mid LAD (arrow)

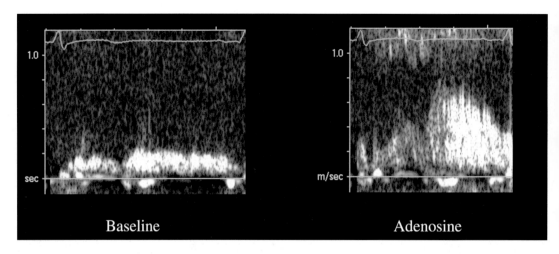

Fig. 53b Transthoracic contrast enhanced PW Doppler: Normal increase of LAD flow during adenosine infusion

change. If during hyperemia the Doppler angle or the LAD segment in the colour image appears different to that visualised at baseline, a new baseline velocity recording should be made in the wash-out phase. This manouvre works better with adenosine because of its rapid reversibility.

3.17.2 Displacement of the sample volume

It is important that a CFR measurement is made in the post-stenotic territory. Post-stenotic CFR is much more accurate than pre-stenotic CFR in assessing the residual vasodilatory capacity of the vascular bed caused by a narrowed coronary artery (68). In fact, coronary flow reserve measured in regions with branches proximal to the lesion is unreliable because flow is concurrently assessed for regions of varying vasodilatatory reserve, so that the result reflects a weighted average of these potentially disparate zones.

The measurement of CFR can also be invalidated if it is taken at the stenosis site itself. Worse still, one can measure blood flow velocity in one segment of the artery at baseline and, with the effect of tachycardia and hyperpnea, in a slightly different segment during hyperemia. If a stenotic jet is inadvertently imaged only during stress, a false-normal CFR can result. To avoid these problems, it is useful at baseline to explore a tract of the artery as long as possible and check that the flow is homogeneous. If abnormally high flow is detected in one portion of the artery, the sample volume should be placed as distally as possible from the stenosis site, making sure that in the new location flow velocity is in the normal range. This position should be maintained throughout the examination.

3.17.3 Flow in the mammary artery

Flow in mammary artery can be mistaken for coronary flow. It can, however, easily be recogn-

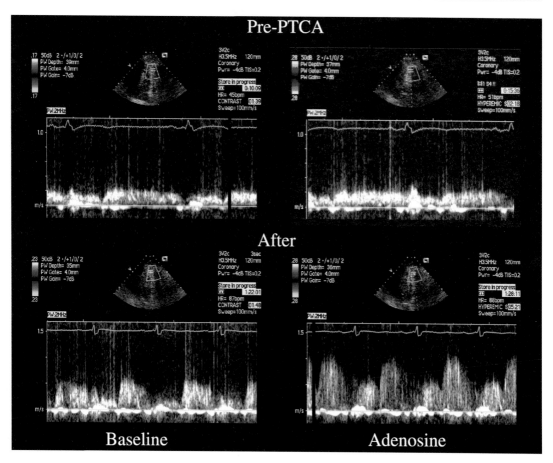

Fig. 54 CFR measurements before and one week after PTCA of a subocclusive proximal LAD stenosis. Before PTCA (top panel) the spectra of LAD flow were flat with a ratio of the systolic to the diastolic velocities of one. Almost no change was found between baseline (left) and adenosine recordings (right). After PTCA (bottom panel) the typical pattern of normal coronary flow is recorded with higher velocities in diastole than in systole.

ised by its lack of cardiac motion and by the prevalent systolic velocity component of its Doppler signal.

3.17.4 Bubble noise

Small bubbles enhance the Doppler signal without affecting the echo statistics, so that the character of the spectral Doppler sound does not change. Larger bubbles, on the other hand, pass through the sensitive volume as single, highly reflective scatterers and create transients which are readily heard as 'popping' sounds. They give rise to the familiar bidirectional 'spike' in the Doppler spectrum (Chapter 1). The same effect is also caused by bubbles which are disrupted by the ultrasound pressure as they pass through the sample volume. Agents such as Levovist, as they disintegrate in the blood stream, appear to aggregate into larger collections of gas, which are capable of

Pitfalls in CFR measurement

Technical problems

- Angle of the vessel to the beam
- Displacement of the sample volume
- Inadvertant scanning of internal mammary artery
- Bubble noise

Interpretation problems

- Impact of preload, blood pressure, vasodilation

producing this artifactual echo appearance in the wash-out phase. The PW Doppler recordings in Figure 55 show the typical spikes of an air based agent which is breaking up as a result of its passage through the heart and lungs. Bubble noise can be avoided by reducing the transmit power (that is the MI, not the gain!).

3.17.5 Interpretation problems: impact of preload

Increase of preload caused by aortic or mitral regurgitation, anemia, high cardiac output, etc. reduces CFR by increasing basal flow through an increase in oxygen consumption. On the other hand, an increased heart rate reduces CFR by increasing basal flow and at same time decreasing maximal flow (69). Thus, any reduction of absolute CFR must always be interpreted in the light of the hemodynamic conditions. A general increase of basal flow velocit, is often detectable in these circumstances.

3.17.6 Impact of blood pressure

Blood pressure has little effect on CFR since alterations in aortic pressure within the limits of autoregulation produce parallel increases in basal and maximal coronary flow, so that CFR remains the same (69). This is true if blood pressure variations affect both baseline and hyperemia in a uniform way. However, a drop in blood pressure can occur only in the hyperemic part of the study as a consequence of the adenosine effect on systemic arterial resistance. When this occurs, even small blood pressure

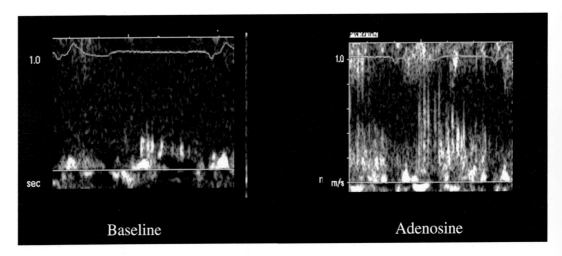

Fig. 55 Bubble noise: the Doppler spectrum is composed of a series of spikes which represent disruption of the microbubbles.

variations can induce large variation of maximal coronary blood flow since, with the removal of autoregulation by adenosine, the relation between blood flow and blood pressure becomes very steep (69). CFR can therefore be affected profoundly by adenosine-induced blood pressure variations. Blood pressure must always be monitored carefully even though significant adenosine-induced blood pressure variation, in our experience, affects less than 10 percent of patients. A variation of more than 30 mm Hg in blood pressure during adenosine with respect to baseline invalidates the CFR measurement.

3.17.7 Vasodilation during hyperemia

One reason for errors in assessing coronary flow reserve with this Doppler method and adenosine could be flow-mediated dilation of the epicardial vessels during hyperemia (70). If this phenomenon should occur, CFR as the simple ratio of two velocities would underestimate true coronary flow reserve, since maximal velocity would be reduced as consequence of vasodilatation. Current knowledge suggests that this effect is limited in patients with arteriosclerosis and intravenous application of adenosine and dipyridamol, but further studies are needed to shed more light on this issue.

3.18 Summary

For echocardiography, contrast agents present a unique opportunity to add assessment of myocardial perfusion to the examination of the patient with ischemic disease. From a technical point of view, the examination is a challenging one which requires both training and experience. There is no question that as the technology of both the contrast agents and the imaging instruments improve, so the examination will become easier to perform. The advent of real-time, low MI perfusion imaging is one of the most significant advances in this regard. Triggered harmonic power Doppler remains the most sensitive available method, but it is hampered by very low framerates and the challenge of recognising and minimising motion artifact. The integration of these techniques with the stress echo is fundamental to its success and initial experience is very promising. There is every reason to expect that real-time contrast perfusion stress echo will be a routine procedure in the near future. Quantitative assessment of coronary flow reserve from contrast enhanced measurement of velocity in apical vessels is a well-validated stress procedure that can provide information that is more limited in anatomic domain but easier to acquire than perfusion imaging. With both these methods, contrast ultrasound offers the opportunity to provide quantitative perfusion information previously unavailable in a simple, real-time procedure.

3.19 References

1. Marcus ML. Anatomy of coronary vasculature. In: Marcus ML (editor) The coronary circulation in health and disease. McGraw Hill, New York 1983: 3–21

2. Myers JH, Stirling MC, Choy M et al. Direct measurement of inner and outer wall thickening dynamics with epicardial echocardiography: Circulation 1986, 74: 164–172

3. Braunwald E, Kloner RA. Myocardial reperfusion: A double-edge sword? J Clin Invest 1985; 76:1715

4. Epstein SE, Cannon RO, Talbot TL. Hemodynamic principles in the control of coronary blood flow. Am J Cardiol 1985; 56:8E

5. Kaul S, Jayaweera AR. Coronary and myocardial blood volumes: noninvasive tools to assess the coronary microcirculation? Circulation 1997; 96: 719–724

6. Wei K, Jayaweera Ar, Firoozan S et al. Quantification of myocardial blood flow using ultrasound-induced destruction of microbubbles administered as a constant venous infusion. Circulation 1998; 97: 473–483

7. Schlant RC, Blomquist CG, Brandenburg RO et al. Guidelines for exercise testing: A report of the Joint American College of Cardiology-American Heart Association Task Force on Assessment of cardiovascular procedures. Circulation 1986; 74 (suppl III):653A

8. Gianrossi R, Detrano R, Mulvihill D et al. Exercise-induced ST depression in the diagnosis of coronary artery disease. A meta analysis. Circulation 1989; 80:87

9. Armstrong WF, Mueller TM, Kinney EL, Tickner EG, Dillon JC, Feigenbaum H. Assessment of myocardial perfusion abnormalities with contrast-enhanced two-dimensional echocardiography. Circulation 1982; 66(1):166–173

10. Marwick TH, Nemecc JJ, Pashkow FJ et al.Accuracy and limitations of exercise echocardiography in a routine clinical setting. J Am Coll Cardiol 1992; 19:74–81

11. Elhendy A, Geleijnse ML, Roelandt JRTC, et al. Dobutamine-induced hypoperfusion without transient wall motion abnormalities: less severe ischemia or less severe stress? J Am Coll Cardiol 1996; 27:323–9

12. Geleijnse ML, Salustri A, Marwick TH et al. Should the diagnosis of coronary artery disease be based on the evaluation of myocardial fucntion or perfusion? Eur Heart J 1997; 18 (suppl D):D68–D77

13. Kaul S. Myocardial contrast echocardiography. 15 years of research and development. Circulation 1997; 96:3745–3760

14. Kaul S, Pandian NG, Okada RD et al. Contrast echocardiography in acute myocardial ischemia: I.In vivo determination of total left ventricular 'area ar risk'. J Am Coll Cardiol 1984; 4:1272–1282

15. Ragosta M, Camarano GP, Kaul S, Powers E, Gimple LW. Microvascular integrity indicates myocellular viability in patients with recent myocardial infarction: new insights using myocardial contrast echocardiography. Circulation 1994; 89:2562–2569

16. Distante A, Rovai D. Stress echocardiography and myocardial contrast echocardiography in viability assessment. European Heart Journal 1997; 18:714–715

17. Sabia PJ, Powers ER, Jayaweera AR, Ragosta M, Kaul S. Functional significance of collateral blood flow in patients with recent myocardial infarction: a study using myocardial contrast echocardiography. Circulation 1992; 85: 2080–2089

18. Cheirif J, Desir RM, Bolli R, Mahmarian JJ, Zoghbi WA, Verani MS, Quinones MA. Relation of perfusion defects observed with myocardial contrast echocardiography to the severity of coronary stenosis: correlation with thallium-201 single-photon emission tomography. J Am Coll Cardiol 1992; 19(6):1343–1349

19. Kaul S, Senior R, Dittrich H, Raval U, Khattar R, Lahiri A. Detection of coronary artery disease with myocardial contrast echocardiography: comparison with 99mTc-sestamibi single-photon emission computed tomography. Circulation 1997; 96(3):785–792

20. Agrawal DI, Malhotra S, Nanda NC, Truffa CC, Agrawal G, Thakur Ac, Jamil F, Taylor GW, Becher H. Harmonic Power Doppler Contrast Echocardiography: Preliminary experimental results. Echocardiography 1997; 14,6:631–635

21. Becher H, Tiemann K, Schlief R, Lüderitz B, Nanda NC. Harmonic Power Doppler Contrast Echocardiography: Preliminary clinical results. Echocardiography 1997; 14,6:637–642

22. Tiemann K, Becher H, Bimmel, Schlief R, Nanda N. Stimulated acoustic emission. Nonbackscatter contrast effect of microbubbles seen with harmonic power Doppler imaging. Echocardiography 1997; 14:65–69

23. Becher H. Power Doppler. In: Rush-Presbyterian-St.Luke's Clinical Use of Contrast Echocardiography. (1998) Am J Cardiol – a continuing education

24. Becher H, Tiemann K, Powers J. Power Harmonic Imaging – clinical application in contrast echocardiography. Medica Mundi 1999; 43(2):26–30

25. Porter TR, Li S, Kilzer K et al. Effect of significant two-vessel versus one-vessel coronary artery stenosis on myocardial contrast effects observed with intermittent harmonic imaging after intravenous contrast injection during dobutamine stress echocardiography. J Am Coll Cardiol 1997; 30:1399–1406

26. Marwick TH, Brunken R, Meland N et al. Accuracy and feasability of contrast echocardiography for detection of perfusion defects in routine practice: comparison with wall motion and technetium-99m sestamibi SPECT. J Am Coll Cardiol 1998; 38,5:1260–1269

27. Hope-Simpson D, Chin CT, Burns PN. Pulse Inversion Doppler: A new method for detecting non-linear echoes from microbubble contrast agents. IEEE Transactions UFFC 1999; 46:376–382

28. Tiemann K, Lohmeier S, Kintz S et al. Real-time contrast echo assessment of myocardial perfusion at low emission power: First experimental and clinical results using power pulse inversion imaging. Echocardiography 1999; 16:799–809

29. Porter TR, Xie F. Transient myocardial contrast after initial exposure to diagnostic ultrasound pressures with minute doses of intravenously injected microbubbles: demonstration and potential mechanisms. Circulation 1995; 92:2391–2395

30. Porter TR, Li S, Jiang L, Grayburn P, Deligonul U. Real-time visualization of myocardial perfusion and wall thickening in human beings with intravenous ultrasonographic contrast and accelerated intermittent harmonic imaging. J Am Soc Echocardiogr 1999; 12(4):266–271.

31. Wei K, Jayaweera AR, Firoozan S et al. Basis for detection of stenosis using venous administration of microbubbles during myocardial contrast echocardiography: bolus or continuous infusion? J Am Coll Cardiol 1998; 32:252–260

32. Albrecht T, Urbank A, Mahler M et al. Prolongation and optimization of Doppler enhancement with a microbubble US contrast agent by using continuous infusion: preliminary experience. Radiology 1998; 207:339–347

33. Miller JJ, Tiemann K, Podell S, Becher H, Doerr Stevens JK, Kuvelas T, Greener Y, Killam AAL, Goenechea J, Dittrich HC. Infusion of Optison for left ventricular opacification and myocardial contrast echocardiography. J Am Soc Echocardiogr 1999 (in press)

34. Wilson RF, Wyche K, Christensen BV et al. Effects of adenosine on human coronary arterial circulation. Circulation 1990; 82:1595–1606

35. Johnston DL, Daley JR, Hodge DO, Hopfenspirger MR, Gibbons RJ. Hemodynamic responses and adverse effects associated with adenosine and dipyridamole pharmacologic stress testing: a comparison in 2000 patients. Mayo Clin Proc 1995; 70: 331–336

36. Wei K, Jayaweera AR, Firoozan S et al. Quantification of myocardial blood flow with ultrasound induced destruction of microbubbles administered as a continuous infusion. Circulation 1998; 97:473–483

37. Ito H, Tomooka T, Sakai N et al. Lack of myocardial perfusion immediately after successful thrombolysis: A predictor of poor recovery of left ventricular function in anterior myocardial infarction. Circulation 1992; 85:1699–1705

38. Agati L, Funaro S, Veneroso G, Lamberti A, Altieri C, Bilotta F, Benedetti G, De Castro S, Autore C, Fedele F. Assessment of myocardial reperfusion after acute myocardial infarction using harmonic power Doppler and Levovist: Intravenous versus intracoronary contrast injection. Eur Heart J 1999; 20 (abstract supplement):362

39. Iliceto S, Galiuto L, Marchese A et al. Functional role of microvascular integrity in patients with infarct-related artery patency after acute myocardial infarction. Eur Heart J 1997; 18:618–624

40. Kloner RA; Ganote CE, Jennings RB. The 'no-reflow' phenomen after tempory coronary occlusion in the dog. J Clin Invest 1974; 54:1496–1508

41. Firschke C, Basini R, Patiga J et al. Contrast echo cardiographic evaluation of myocardial salvage after reperfusion therapy in acute myocardial infarction. Eur Heart J 1999; 20 (abstract supplement):363

42. Horcher J, Blasini R, Martinoff S, Schwaiger M, Schömig A, Firschke C. Myocardial perfusion in acute coronary syndrome. Circulation1999; 99:e1

43. Firschke C, Lindner JR, Wei K, Goodman NC, Skyba DM, Kaul S. Myocardial perfusion imaging in the setting of coronary artery stenosis and acute myocardial infarction using venous injection of a second-generation echocardiographic contrast agent. Circulation 1997; 96(3):959–967.

44. Macioch JE, Sandelski J, Ostoic TA, Johnson MS, In M, Thew ST, Liebson PR, Becher H, Holoviak M, Feinstein SB. Clinically reproducible myocardial perfusion studies with contrast echo in 82 consecutive patients:correlation to cardiac cath or nuclear imaging in 36 patients. Echocardiography 1998;15[6, part2]:98

45. Porter TR, Xie F, Kilzer K, Deligonul U. Detection of myocardial perfusion abnormalities during dobutamine and adenosine stress echocardiography with transient myocardial contrast imaging after minute quantities of intravenous perfluorocarbon-exposed sonicated dextrose albumin. J Am Soc Echocardiogr 1996; 9(6):779–786

46. Porter TR, Li S, Kricsfeld D, Armbruster RW. Detection of myocardial perfusion in multiple echocardiographic windows with one intravenous injection of microbubbles using transient response second harmonic imaging. J Am Coll Cardiol 1997; 29(4):791-799.

47. Firschke C. Venous myocardial contrast echocardiography can guide clinical decision making in the catheterization laboratory. Circulation 1998;

48. Lentz C, Tiemann, K, Köster J, Schlosser T, Goenechea J, Becher H. Does color blooming limitate assessment of myocardial perfusion using harmonic power Doppler? Eur Heart J 1999; 20 (abstract supplement):359

49. Gould KL, Lipscomb K, Hamilton GW. Physiologic basis for assessing critical coronary stenosis. Instantaneous flow response and regional distribution during coronary hyperemia as measures of coronary flow reserve. Am.J.Cardiol. 1974; 33:87-94.

50. Doucette JW, Corl PD, Payne HM, Flynn AE, Goto M, Nassi M, Segal J. Validation of a Doppler guide wire for intravascular measurement of coronary artery flow velocity. Circulation 1992; 85:1899-1911.

51. Demer LL, Gould KL, Goldstein RA, Kirkeeide RL, Mullani NA, Smalling RW, Nishikawa A, Merhige ME. Assessment of coronary artery disease severity by positron emission tomography. Comparison with quantitative arteriography in 193 patients. Circulation 1989; 79:825-835

52. Iliceto S, Marangelli V, Memmola C, Rizzon P. Transesophageal Doppler echocardiography evaluation of coronary blood flow velocity in baseline conditions and during dipyridamole-induced coronary vasodilation. Circulation 1991; 83:61-69

53. Iliceto S, Caiati C, Aragona P, Verde R, Schlief R, Rizzon P. Improved Doppler signal intensity in coronary arteries after intravenous peripheral injection of a lung-crossing contrast agent (SHU 508A) . J.Am.Coll.Cardiol. 1994; 23:184-190.

54. Caiati C, Aragona P, Iliceto S, Rizzon P. Improved Doppler detection of proximal left anterior descending coronary artery stenosis after intravenous injection of a lung-crossing contrast agent: a transesophageal Doppler echocardiographic study. J.Am.Coll.Cardiol. 1996; 27:1413-1421

55. Powers JE, Burns PN, Souquet J. Imaging instrumentation for ultrasound contrast agents. In: Nanda NC, Schlief R, Goldberg BB, eds. Advances in echo imaging using contrast enhancement. Kluwer Academic Publishers, 1997:139-170

56. Caiati C, Montaldo C, Zedda N, Bina A, Iliceto S. New noninvasive method for coronary flow reserve assessment: contrast-enhanced transthoracic second harmonic echo Doppler. Circulation 1999; 99:771-778.

57. Lambertz H, Tries HP, Stein T, Lethen H. Noninvasive assessment of coronary flow reserve with transthoracic signal-enhanced Doppler echocardiography. J.Am.Soc.Echocardiogr. 1999; 12:186-195.

58. Mulvagh SL, Foley DA, Aeschbacher BC, Klarich KK, Seward JB. Second harmonic imaging of an intravenously administered echocardiographic contrast agent: Visualization of coronary arteries and measurement of coronary blood flow. J.Am.Coll.Cardiol. 1996; 27:1519-1525.

59. Caiati C, Montaldo C, Zedda N, Montisci R, Ruscazio M, Lai G, Cadeddu M, Meloni L, Iliceto S. Validation of a new non-invasive method (contrast-enhanced transthoracic second harmonic echo Doppler) for the evaluation of coronary flow reserve. Comparison with intra-coronary Doppler flow wire. J.Am.Coll.Cardiol. 1999; 34:1193-1200

60. Caiati C, Zedda N, Montaldo C, Montisci R, Iliceto S. Contrast-enhanced transthoracic second harmonic echo Doppler with adenosine: a non-invasive, rapid and effective method for coronary flow reserve assessment. J.Am.Coll.Cardiol. 1999; 34:122-130.

61. Gould KL, Martucci JP, Goldberg DI, Hess MJ, Edens RP, Latifi R, Dudrick SJ. Short-term cholesterol lowering decreases size and severity of perfusion abnormalities by positron emission tomography after dipyridamole in patients with coronary artery disease. A potential noninvasive marker of healing coronary endothelium. Circulation 1994; 89:1530-1538.

62. Arora GD, Reeves WC, Movahed A. Alteration of coronary perfusion reserve in hypertensive patients with diabetes. J.Hum.Hypertens. 1994; 8:51-57.18

63. Pitkänen OP, Nuutila P, Raitakari OT, Rönnemaa T, Koskinen PJ, Iida H, Lehtimäki TJ, Laine HK, Takala T, Viikari JS, Knuuti J. Coronary flow reserve is reduced in young men with IDDM. Diabetes 1998; 47:248-254.

64. Rossen JD, Quillen JE, Lopez AG, Stenberg RG, Talman CL, Winniford MD. Comparison of coronary vasodilation with intravenous dipyridamole and adenosine. J.Am.Coll.Cardiol. 1991; 18:485-491

65. White CW, Wright CB, Doty DB, Hiratza LF, Eastham CL, Harrison DG, Marcus ML. Does visual

interpretation of the coronary arteriogram predict the physiologic importance of a coronary stenosis? N.Engl.J.Med. 1984; 310:819–824

66. Kern MJ, Donohue TJ, Aguirre FV, Bach RG, Caracciolo EA, Wolford T, Mechem CJ, Flynn MS, Chaitman B. Clinical outcome of deferring angioplasty in patients with normal translesional pressure-flow velocity measurements. J.Am.Coll.Cardiol. 1995; 25:178–187.

67. Wilson RF, Johnson MR, Marcus ML, Aylward PE, Skorton DJ, Collins S, White CW. The effect of coronary angioplasty on coronary flow reserve. Circulation 1988; 77:873–885.

68. Donohue TJ, Kern MJ, Aguirre FV, Bach RG, Wolford T, Bell CA, Segal J. Assessing the hemodynamic significance of coronary artery stenoses: analysis of translesional pressure-flow velocity relations in patients. J.Am.Coll.Cardiol. 1993; 22:449–458.

69. McGinn AL, White CW, Wilson RF. Interstudy variability of coronary flow reserve. Influence of heart rate, arterial pressure, and ventricular preload. Circulation 1990; 81:1319–1330.

70. Takeuchi M, Nohtomi Y, Kuroiwa A. Does coronary flow reserve assessed by blood flow velocity analysis reflect absolute coronary flow reserve? [see comments]. Cathet.Cardiovasc.Diagn. 1996; 38:251–254.

4 Methods for quantitative Analysis

Wann überhaupt, wenn nicht jetzt?
(When at all, if not now?)

Albert Einstein, 1879–1955

Introduction*

It is known that the strength of the echo enhancement in a region perfused by blood carrying microbubbles is approximately proportional to the number of bubbles present. Though attenuation and other technical factors preclude estimation of the absolute concentration of bubbles from the echo amplitude alone, relative changes in bubble concentration in a region of the image can be estimated from the echo signal itself. Knowing this value enables a number of important clinical and physiological estimates to be made, including those of ejection fraction, relative vascular volume, flow velocity and relative perfusion rate. Quantitative reporting of contrast echo studies is likely to become as routine a part of the examination as it is in nuclear medicine.

Today, as contrast echocardiography continues to gain clinical acceptance, the interpretation of images remains essentially qualitative. Techniques for deriving quantitative information from contrast studies are still primarily used in the research rather than the clinical setting (1–5). Hesitation to use image processing in contrast echo may reflect its lack of role in other applications of echocardiography. Until recently, contrast echo image processing has required the use of a video frame grabber and custom designed computer software and hardware. Common difficulties such as off-line videotape transfer, calibration, data compression, and lack of a standard computer operating system has limited its clinical potential. Therefore, users of myocardial contrast echo may be resistant to perform time-consuming off-line analysis and therefore confine themselves to visual judgement of unprocessed recordings.

In response to the need for accessible image processing for clinical contrast echocardiography, several commercially available software packages have emerged from, among others, Sklenar at the University of Virginia, ATL Ultrasound, Agilent and GE/Vingmed. These packages are either integrated into the ultrasound systems or use standard personal computer (PC) hardware, and comprise basic software routines which allows users to analyse contrast echo information quickly. Although image processing may at first appear intimidating, the basic operations when taken singly are easy to learn and perform.

4.1 Basic tools for image quantification

The simplest form of contrast echo analysis requires only a single image, for example to measure a cavity volume or compare enhancement in different regions of the myocardium. Following the time course of enhancement needs cineloop analysis; this also forms the basis of flow calculations in myocardial perfusion studies.

Basic tools used in contrast echo image processing range from simple drawing and statistical calculations to sophisticated editing, image alignment, and graphing tools, all of which are aimed at measuring the effect of the contrast agent on the backscattered signal from blood. These tools are applied sequentially to single frames or to series of frames (cineloops). Therefore, learning the steps involved is as simple a becoming familiar some basic tools, and a flowchart for their use.

*This section courtesy of Danny M Skyba and Damien Dolimier, Bothell WA, USA

Quantitative Methods

4.1.1 Single image quantification

After selecting a representative contrast enhanced frame, the user may select a pixel location ('Pick'), draw a region-of-interest (ROI) encompassing an area, or select a linear ROI or 'Profile'. Figure 1 shows a single image along with the results generated by a 'pick' and a ROI. The result of a pick or ROI is typically the intensity value of the pixel selected, or the mean intensity of the pixels contained within the ROI. For a profile, a vector or graph of intensities along the line is displayed. Intensity data within a ROI can also be displayed as an array of information or as a histogram, rather than as a single mean intensity. Figure 1 shows examples of these data.

Steps involved in processing single image

1. Select a representative frame
2. Select the desired tool for collecting intensity information, such as a 'pick', 'profile', ROI or histogram
3. Draw or 'pick' a region or pixel
4. Display and interpret the resulting amplitude data
5. Repeat for different regions in the image, if desired

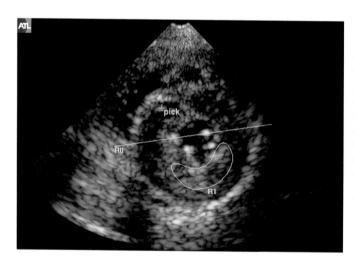
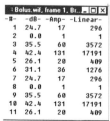
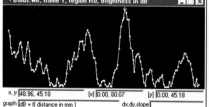
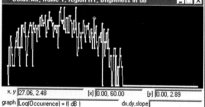

'pick list'   profile along R0   histogram in R1

Fig. 1 Analysis of a single image selected from a cineloop. Four different regions have been drawn in the image: a pick region, a line (R0), and a free-form ROI (R1). Below are examples of results which can be generated using single frame quantification. The pick result is a dynamic statistical list to which entries are added each time as user 'picks' a pixel. A profile is generated along the line (R0). A histogram displays the amplitude data in the free-form ROI (R1).

4.1.2 Cineloop quantification

Although single image quantification may allow a user to determine and compare intensity values between various myocardial beds or chambers, temporal information is ignored. Since ultrasound is a real-time imaging modality, it is the interpretation of image intensity data as a function of time that forms the basis for the quantification of myocardial perfusion from contrast echo images. Fortunately, quantification of an entire cineloop of images is not much more difficult than that of a single image. Time behaviour of a bolus is one aspect of a contrast study that can be analysed using such an approach.

Prior to processing cineloop data, the user must review the images carefully and take note of the quality of the images and the data. Does the loop capture the information required? Is the image size and quality satisfactory? Are there artifacts or other image frames which need to be excluded? Which frame is best suited for placement of a representative ROI? Quick mental notes during review can save lots of time during the editing, quantification and data interpretation steps that follow. Additionally, if the user performing the analysis has different image preferences from the sonographer, aesthetic information such as the grey map and colour map can often be changed without changing the underlying intensity data. This can be especially beneficial in creating results that are similar in presentation to those of nuclear cardiology images. If the data analysis is not performed immediately during the echo exam, information regarding the patient is usually stored within the image files and can be used later to organise stages of a study.

4.1.2.1 Reduction of data

The first step in quantifying a cineloop information is to reduce the data. Usually, many more images are collected during the ultrasound examination than are required for analysis. Data reduction speeds up image quantitation routines and also prevents artifactual data from being displayed as a result. Simple software editing tools allow the user to select a new first and last frame in the cineloop for processing. Additionally, the user may single out individual image frames and 'cut' them out of the loop. Frames containing image artifacts such as ectopic beats or post-extrasystolic beats should be excluded, as should frames with severe wall motion artifacts. Other common artifacts include arrhythmias, exaggerated patient breathing, momentarily poor transducer contact or unwanted transducer translation. ECG information is often included in the cineloop allowing the user to justify data reduction.

4.1.2.2 Positioning Regions of Interest (ROI)

Once relevant image frames have been selected, the next processing step is to specify a ROI within which measurements will be made. A representative frame in the cineloop is selected and the user may choose a particular shape, or create a custom ROI. ROIs are often drawn using the standard segmental model of the American Society of Echocardiography. One ROI should be placed within a single segment or perfusion territory, and the size of the ROI should cover most of the segment. ROIs within a segment should be as large as possible to minimise statistical error within the ROI, as well as to reduce scatter of the single measurements for consecutive frames (6). To minimise tedium, the ROI is usually drawn only once in the representative frame, and is automatically applied to the same position in every cineloop frame.

It is important that the cineloop be reviewed to validate the position of every ROI in each frame to be evaluated. The borders of the ROIs must not touch the endocardial borders, otherwise the measurements in the ROI may be corrupted by the strong contrast signals within the cavity. ROIs which 'fall out' of the myocardium and into the LV cavity will skew the mean intensity value for that frame. To correct ROI position problems, image alignment must be performed. The specific methods used for image alignment differ among the software available, but options for image or region adjustment are generally available. The first option is image alignment, where the position of the cineloop images can be changed to match the position of the fixed ROI. (Figure 2) This is the traditional method of correcting for heart motion and translation in contrast echo image analysis (7–8). The second option is ROI adjustment, where the ROI can be individually repositioned in each frame to match the anatomy of the unaligned images (Figure 3). When these operations are performed man-

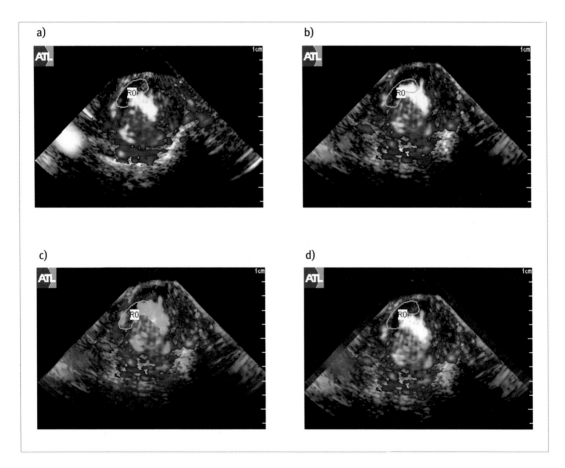

Fig. 2 (a) Reference image with a well positioned ROI. (b) Unaligned frame with the ROI falling into the LV cavity. (c) The user performs manual alignment by positioning the unaligned frame (green) over the reference frame (magenta). (d) Optimal alignment is indicated by a mostly grey image.

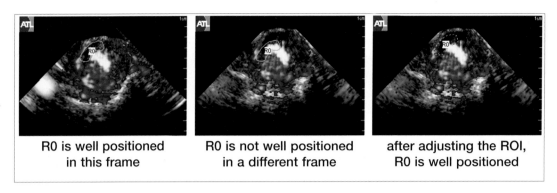

| R0 is well positioned in this frame | R0 is not well positioned in a different frame | after adjusting the ROI, R0 is well positioned |

Fig. 3 The same case as Figure 2 where the user repositions the ROI in each frame so that the ROI represents the same anatomic region. In the case of ROI adjustment, the new ROI appears dashed, indicating that it has been repositioned; further editing of the ROI is performed on a frame-by-frame basis.

ually, both are equally reliable in correcting for simple motion, such as in plane movement of the sonographers hand position. When tracking an ROI over the entire cardiac cycle, ROI adjustment is preferable, since image alignment is difficult with dynamically changing images. In contrast, when images are triggered at a particular phase of the cardiac cycle, such as end systole or end diastole, manual image alignment may be faster. Image alignment also allows placement of multiple ROIs and aligns the image only once for all ROIs.

4.1.2.3 Automatic analysis

Some software packages offer options for automatic image alignment using cross-correlation techniques. If available, automatic alignment routines should be tried first. When successful, automatic alignment algorithms greatly speed data analysis. An advantage of image processing software packages which capture direct digital data rather than frame grabbed intensity data is that colour ultrasound information can be accurately quantified. Because of the improved segmentation provided by colour imaging techniques, harmonic power Doppler (HPD) images may be superior to B-mode greyscale images in delineating myocardium from LV cavity in contrast frames. This difference can be visually appreciated using a colour-coded display which is already implemented on commercially available ultrasound systems. High power signals originate from contrast within the cavities and are displayed in a single bright colour when they reach a variable threshold. Low power signals are caused by contrast within the myocardium. Different hues of a complementary colour provide the visual information on the concentration of microbubbles in the sample volume. This segmentation of the LV cavity from the myocardium can facilitate ROI placement. The contrast in colour along the border of the LV also provides an excellent 'edge' for cross-correlation based alignment techniques. Unfortunately, without some additional post-processing, some users of HPD techniques report 'bleeding' intensity signal from the LV cavity into the myocardium which may result in artificially high myocardial intensity data. These users prefer to operate on B-mode greyscale images where ROI placement and image alignment must often be performed manually, and cautiously.

The final step in basic image processing of cineloops is to quantify and display the data. In the case of a ROI, it is the mean image intensity contained within the ROI that is plotted for every frame in the cineloop, usually as a function of time. Software that requires calibration takes this into account at the time of result calculation. Software packages that are integrated into ultrasound hardware, or use proprietary image formats perform internal calibration automatically. Tools for rescaling data results are also generally available.

Steps involved in processing cineloops:

1. Load and review the cineloop visually. Note the need for loop editing and alignment
2. Edit the cineloop by selecting new first and last frames (if necessary)
3. Remove individual frames from the cineloop that may contain artifacts
4. Select a representative frame from the cineloop
5. Draw one or more ROIs on the image in the desired perfusion territories
6. Visually review the edited cineloop, carefully noting the position of the ROI(s) in each frame
7. Align the images or the individual ROIs. Try automatic routines (if available) before resorting to manual alignment
8. Review aligned ROIs. Re-adjust individual ROIs manually if necessary
9. Display and scale the results

4.2 Advanced image processing: cases & examples

The current state-of-the-art for advanced processing of contrast echocardiographic images is really nothing more than a combination of basic image processing routines with a few technical and mathematical enhancements. In this section, we describe some commonly employed routines through a series of experimental and clinical examples.

4.2.1 Single image quantification

The simplest form of quantification is on a single still image taken from a cineloop. Typically, a single representative frame can be chosen from a baseline cineloop, where a patient is at rest, and another image can be taken from a cineloop during peak stress. Visually disparate information between the two images can be validated quantitatively by measuring intensity levels in various perfusion beds before and after stress. The tools of choice in this case are the intensity 'pick', or the ROI tool with comparison of the mean image intensity under the ROI. Figure 4a shows normal myocardium at rest. Two regions have been carefully selected in the LAD and LCx beds, respectively, and pick results as well as the mean intensity under the ROI is shown for both ROIs. In Figure 4b, a moderate stenosis has been applied to the LCx. The same ROIs have been overlaid on this image and the pick and mean intensity values are shown. In this simple case, it is visually apparent that there is a lack of contrast in the region supplied by the stenosed LCx. The statistical information provided by the image processing software provides a means of putting a value on the decrease in intensity. In experimental models, it has been shown that the normalised decrease in intensity can be correlated to a decrease in myocardial flow. Therefore, in the case of a mild stenosis or where visual information is not as clear in the example given here, computer

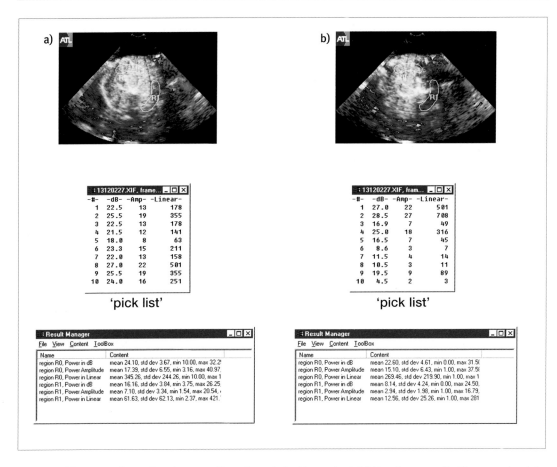

Fig. 4 (a) A normally perfused myocardium. A statistical intensity 'pick' has been applied to several points in both beds, and the results are displayed in the window. A simple ROI has also been drawn and the mean intensity for both beds is shown in the window (in dB, amplitude and linear scales). (b) The same myocardial plane with a moderate stenosis in the LCx bed. The results show a decrease in 'pick' and mean intensity

aided statistical processing offers a method for approximate assessment of perfusion.

4.2.2 Background subtraction

The use of background subtraction has been championed by Kaul, et. al. since the earliest days of contrast echocardiographic image processing (7–8). While the concept is not difficult to understand, it is very important if harmonic B-mode or pulse inversion are used for imaging the myocardium. This is because the level of contrast enhancement at high MI is often only a few decibels above the background level created by the tissue harmonic. Subtraction assumes that image signal other than the enhancement due to the contrast agent is 'background' information, or noise. Additionally, the amount of background information, or noise-floor, may change slightly due to subtle changes in the position of the transducer during an echo examination. Since the only signal of interest is that due to the agent, the background intensity information is subtracted from the total signal and discarded. When this concept is applied to the B-mode image, areas of increased perfusion appear brighter, while areas which lack perfusion, hence contrast enhancement, appear darker. Since the signal due to the contrast may be subtle, this simple technique provides the clinical reader with an enhanced visual perception of perfusion (Figure 5).

In practice background subtraction should always be performed with multiple image groups where the result of the subtraction is, more or less, an average subtracted image. All images should be acquired at the same point in the cardiac cycle and they should be divided into two groups of three or more images: the background group and the contrast-enhanced group. For each pixel position within a group, an image is created containing mean intensity per pixel position. Then the mean values of the two groups are subtracted as shown above, on a pixel by pixel basis. An example of this is shown in Figure 6. Figure 6a shows three pre-contrast images and the mean pre-contrast image. Figure 6b shows three post-contrast images and the mean post-contrast image. Figure 6c shows the result of the subtraction of the pre-contrast image from the post-contrast image, where the intensity is primarily attributed to contrast agent. In this single image we have captured only the information of primary interest, thus making a more rapid interpretation possible. When combined with curve-fitting techniques, the technique of background subtraction provides the data for the statistical analysis of perfusion.

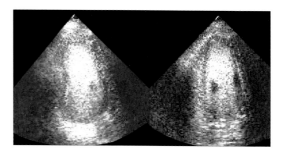

Fig. 5 (a) 44-year old woman with infero-lateral MI who underwent obtuse marginal branch PTCA. (b) Subtracted contrast images show improved perfusion in the infero-posterior wall following PTCA. *Courtesy of Thomas Marwick and Brian Haluska, University of Brisbane, Australia*

Figure 7 shows an example of automated post processing used to evaluate adenosine induced changes in myocardial perfusion volume in a patient with a 99 percent left anterior descending artery lesion. After recording pre- and post-adenosine baseline images (Figure 7a, b), the analysis software performs automatic alignment of the images combined to produce averaged images (Figure 7c, d). Some reduction in image intensity, representing a reduction in myocardial blood volume and redistribution of myocardial perfusion is seen at the apex. The post adenosine averaged image is subtracted from the post adenosine image and the resulting difference displayed with a colour map (Figure 7e). Since the acquired images have logarithmic grey scales, the effect of subtraction is to display their ratio. Myocardial segments that are perfused by coronary beds with good flow reserve should increase in myocardial blood volume following adenosine and are shown in red shades. Segments supplied by diseased vessels become relatively underperfused and the resulting reduction is colour coded blue. In practice, adenosine can cause a hyperventilatory response in some patients which can make image acquisition difficult.

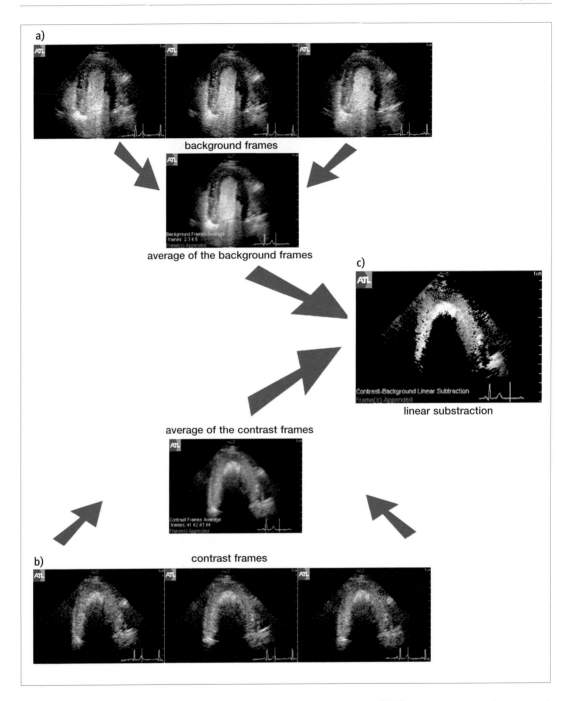

Fig. 6 (a) Three pre-contrast images and the mean pre-contrast image. (b) Three post-contrast images and the mean post-contrast image. (c) The result of the subtraction of the pre-contrast image from the post-contrast. The technique has reduced the amount of background 'noise' and highlights the intensity attributed to contrast agent.

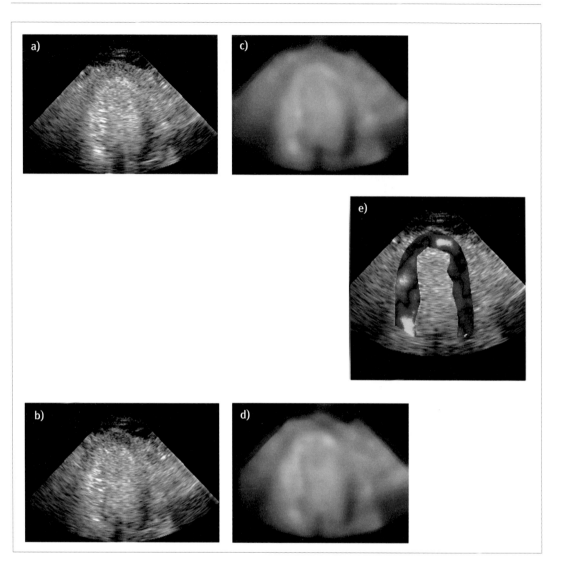

Fig. 7 Post processing used to evaluate adenosine induced changes in myocardial perfusion volume in a patient with a 99 percent left anterior descending artery lesion. End systolic, 2 beat interval intermittent, pulse inversion images are acquired during an injection of Sonazoid before (a) and after (b) a short adenosine infusion. The images are transferred to an off-line workstation for processing using software developed by Dr Morten Eriksen (Nycomed Amersham), which performs automatic alignment of the images which are averaged to produce pre- (c) and post- (d) adenosine images. Some reduction in image intensity, representing a reduction in myocardial blood volume and redistribution of myocardial perfusion is seen at the apex. The post adenosine averaged image is subtracted from the post adenosine image and the resulting difference displayed in colour (e). Since the acquired images have logarithmic grey scales, the effect of subtraction is to display their ratio. Good flow reserve areas give high signal ratios and are shown in red; poor flow reserve areas with low ratios are shown in blue.
Courtesy of Mark J Monaghan, King's College Hospital, London, UK and Morten Eriksen, Nycomed Amersham, Oslo, Norway.

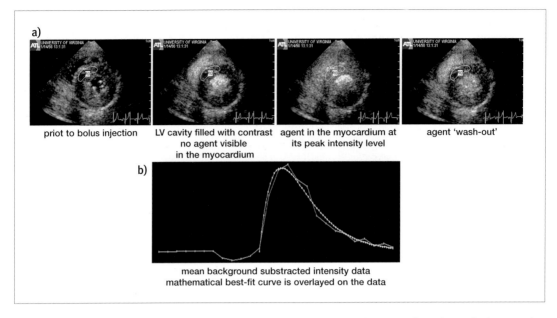

Fig. 8 (a) A series of four images taken in time sequence from a cineloop. The first shows the image prior to bolus injection. The second shows the LV cavity filled with contrast, but no agent is visible in the myocardium. The third image shows the agent in the myocardium at its peak intensity level. Image four shows the slowly decreasing intensity level as the agent 'washes-out' of the vascular system. (b) The mean background subtracted intensity data from the ROI corresponding to all end-systolic images in the cineloop. The mathematical best-fit curve is overlayed on the data.

However, this technique clearly shows the potential of the combination of three new technologies: adenosine echo contrast perfusion, pulse inversion imaging and colour-coded subtraction post processing.

4.2.3 Analysing the time-course of enhancement

4.2.3.1 Intravenous bolus technique

Tracking changes in the intensity level due to contrast agents over the time-course of a bolus injection yields information which is related to the flow of blood to the myocardium (8–10). While deriving information by visually tracking the intensity due to a bolus is difficult, computer aided image processing and statistical curve-fitting are well suited to this task. The result of computed curve-fitting is a single parameter which in certain circumstances can be related to the perfusion rate of blood to the myocardium.

The technique is usually performed as follows. Real-time information in the form of cineloop of images is acquired just prior to, and during the injection of a rapid bolus of contrast agent. Figure 8a shows a series of four images taken in sequence from a cineloop during this time course. The first shows the image prior to bolus injection. The second shows the LV cavity filled with contrast, with no agent is visible in the myocardium. The third image shows the agent in the myocardium at its peak intensity level, and the fourth shows the slowly decreasing intensity levels as the agent washes out of the vascular system. Figure 8b shows the data as a series of points taken from the full cineloop of information. Each data point is the mean intensity under the ROI for each frame of the cineloop. In this example, the data were reduced so that only end-systolic frames are shown. Each data point is subtracted from the level of background intensity, taken as an average of a few representative frames prior to the injection of contrast. The data usually are then fitted to a curve predicted by a model such as the gamma-variate model. This process reduces the data to only two parameters: the amplitude scale and the mean-transit time. The mean transit time has been shown to correlate closely with myocardial flow in experimental models under very specific conditions and may therefore be relevant to clinical perfusion studies. Many commercial image processing packages have the provision for this curve-fitting procedure. However, a number of difficulties with this technique, especially the lack of knowledge of the precise form of the bolus that enters the myocardial bed, limit its usefulness in clinical practice, for which the negative bolus method offers many advantages.

4.2.3.2 Negative bolus technique
Principles
In this technique, a continuous infusion of contrast agent during intermittent triggered

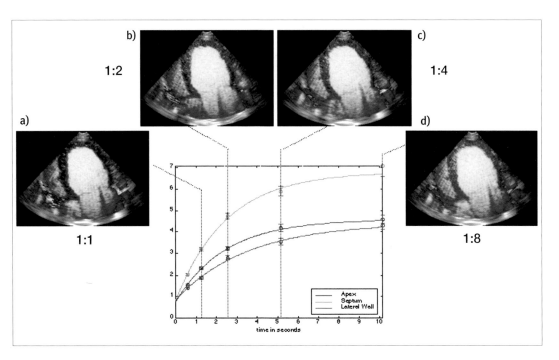

Fig. 9 Negative bolus destruction-reperfusion study using harmonic power Doppler. Regions of interest are placed in the apex, lateral wall and septum and repeated measurements made at each of 1, 2, 4 and 8 heartbeat intervals. The graph shows reperfusion curves for each area. All fit well to a monoexponential function, as predicted by the model described in the text.

imaging is used to overcome the limitations of the bolus injection model. The method is based on the simple principle of *destruction-reperfusion* (11,12). The transducer is positioned over the region of interest in the myocardium and a steady infusion of the agent is established. Using ECG-gated, high MI imaging in harmonic power Doppler mode, a series of perfusion images is made of the myocardium. At one trigger per heartbeat, these images will reflect the amount of blood that has reperfused the myocardium in a single heartbeat (Figure 9 a). If the interval is increased to two heartbeats, a higher intensity is seen as bubbles from smaller vessels refill the myocardium after each disruptive pulse (Figure 8 b). At a four beat interval, the echo level of the myocardium increases more (Figure 9 c). By an eight beat interval, the myocardium attains its maximal brightness, because sufficient time has passed for all bubbles, even those moving most slowly, to refill the myocardium (Figure 9 d). It can readily be appreciated that the brightness of the final image reflects the total number of bubbles present in the region of interest (the total vascular volume), whereas the rate at which this level is attained reflects the speed (or mean velocity) of flow into the region. The product of these two quantities is the flow or perfusion rate. By plotting the mean echo level against time (Figure 9 e), the flowrate can be estimated by fitting a simple exponential curve. The principle is identical to that of indicator dilution theory used in, for

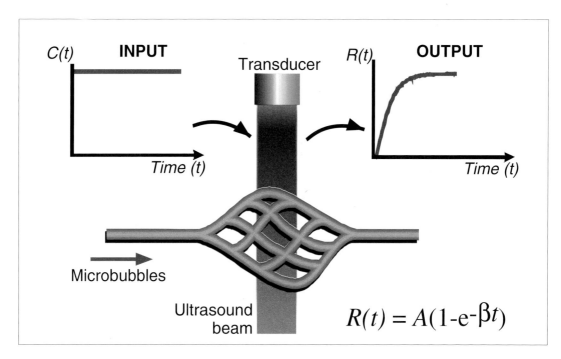

Fig. 10 Principle of negative bolus (or *destruction-reperfusion*) indicator dilution measurement. During a steady infusion of agent, the bubbles are disrupted in the scan plane. The rate at which they wash back in to the image plane is proportional to flow rate. The relative number of bubbles present at incremental intervals from disruption is measured by a further imaging frame, triggered to occur at varying times after the destruction. Real-time power pulse inversion imaging can image the reperfusion process in real time.

example, the thermodilution calculation of cardiac output, but here the bolus is the destruction of the agent, hence the name of the technique. It should be noted that because the echo level from the region of interest is influenced by quantities other than the bubble number (for example, the cavity attenuation), this method only yields a relative flow value. Figure 10 shows the principle of the method and the results of mathematical analysis of the bolus behaviour. Analysis of a negative bolus study is straightforward: all that is required is to find the asymptotic (that is the plateau) value (A) of the enhancement following reperfusion, and the exponent (β) of a simple exponential function fitted to the reperfusion curve. The value A is related to the vascular volume, the value β to the reperfusion velocity. Their product yields an estimate of relative perfusion rate.

Clinical technique
Using a steady infusion, ECG gated images are acquired at different triggering intervals on the ultrasound system. Individual images in the cineloop can be grouped according to the triggering interval. A ROI is positioned as pre-

Negative bolus measurement of myocardial perfusion

1. Establish an infusion and set up imaging (see §1.2.3)
2. Acquire a set of images at each trigger interval
3. Freeze and store image data
4. Position ROI in myocardium and review to ensure that cavity is excluded
5. Plot reperfusion curve and use analysis software to fit exponential
6. Compare exponent (related to velocity) and asymptote (related to volume) between regions of interest

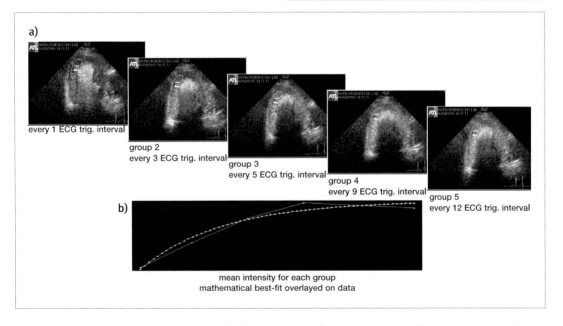

Fig. 11 Negative bolus destruction-reperfusion study using harmonic B-mode. Five representative frames are taken at every 1, 3, 5, 9 and 12 ECG triggering intervals (a). The grouped and averaged data from the entire cineloop are shown in (b) with the mathematical best-fit.

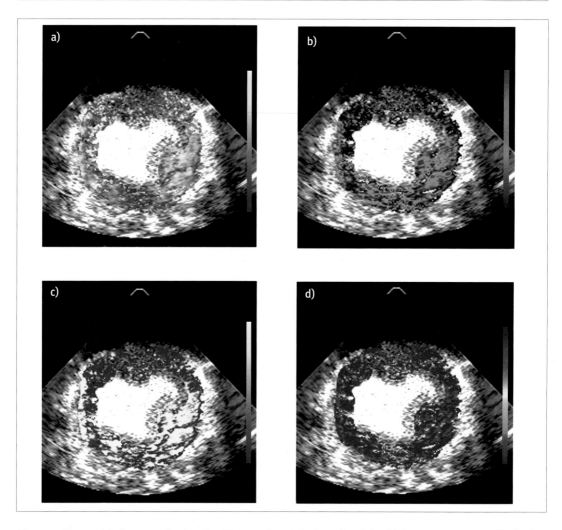

Fig. 12 Parametric images of a heart with experimental stenosis of the LAD coronary artery, displaying calculated parameters from the negative bolus method. These 'parametric' images show (a) Blood volume, (b) blood velocity, (c) blood flow and (d) goodness of fit of the exponential model. Images were digitised from video tape, selected, aligned, averaged, and masked. Then an exponential function was fitted for every selected pixel and parameters defining the local best fit curve displayed using different colour maps.
Courtesy of Jiri Sklenar, University of Virginia, USA. Processing was done on a Macintosh PC using software developed at the University of Virginia and by Yabko, LLC.

viously described, and the mean intensity data is averaged with data from within its group. Curve fitting is then performed, using a monoexponential function. Mathematically, the technique is appealing since all of the pertinent information can be captured with a single expression containing three variables: the background intensity level (the constant), the rate of rise (the initial slope), and a final asymptotic value (the plateau). It has been shown that the slope may relate to the rate of reperfusion of the myocardium after contrast destruction by

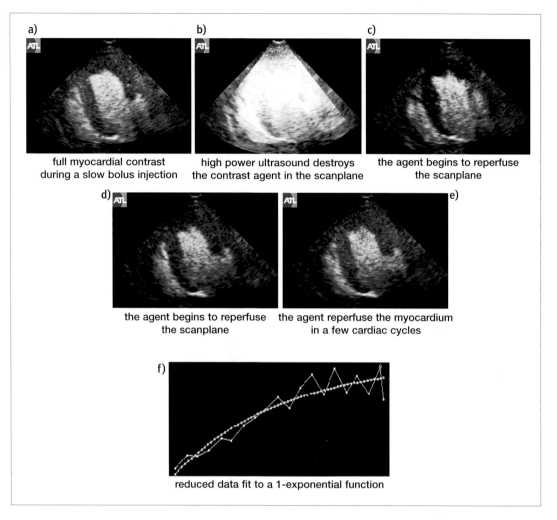

Fig. 13 Real-time myocardial contrast during a slow bolus injection at low MI using Power Pulse Inversion imaging (a). High power frames destroy all of the contrast agent in the scanplane (b). The agent begins to reperfuse the scanplane (c–d), and fully reperfuses the myocardium in a few cardiac cycles (e). Real-time data collection begins just after the high power frames. The data is reduced to include only end diastolic frames, and a monoexponential curve is fitted (f).

ultrasound, and that the plateau value may relate to the volume of the myocardial bed. Figure 11 illustrates this type of analysis performed on harmonic B-mode images. Figure 12 shows how the processing can be taken a step further, producing parametric images whose colours display the quantities calculated by the model. These include relative blood volume, blood velocity and relative blood flow. An image can also be made (Figure 12 d) showing the extent to which the data conform to the model.

4.2.3.3 Real-time negative bolus technique

The new ultrasound technology of power pulse inversion (see §1.3.3.6) allows the rate of reperfusion of contrast to be determined in real-time, rather than with intermittent triggered imaging. The scanner is set to image continuously at low MI (typically 0.1 or less). The trigger then determines the point at which a single burst of high MI frames are introduced to disrupt the bubbles. Reperfusion is then imaged continuously at low MI. Figure 13 shows the real-time reperfusion of contrast into the myocardium after such a series of high MI frames have disrupted all of the contrast agent in the scanplane. The monoexponential function is applied to the entire data set, or to the reduced data. Because it works in real-time, this quantitative method is most likely to evolve into technique integrated into a scanner's software.

4.3 Summary

As the importance of contrast ultrasound grows in the field of cardiology, so will the need for automated routines to provide robust and consistent data to the cardiologist. Based on the interest and investment in the field of contrast echocardiography, it appears likely that the image processing routines discussed here will soon become incorporated into the daily routine of the clinical lab. The importance of providing the research clinician with a user-friendly set of tools can be appreciated. Simultaneously, research in contrast echocardiography is still evolving rapidly. The software developed for contrast echo must have the capacity for future enhancement and expansion. Fortunately, this type of growth can be provided through the use of expandable software modules. Tools are likely to mature to the point that they will be simple to use, standardised and perhaps seamlessly incorporated into ultrasound systems themselves, graduating finally from their modest origins in an off-line personal computer.

4.4 References

1. Ong K, Maurer G, Feinstein S, Zwehl W, Meerbaum S, Corday E. Computer methods for myocardial contrast two-dimensional echocardiography. J Am Coll Cardiol 1984; 3:1212–1218.

2. Skorton DJ, Collins SM, Garcia E, Geiser EA, Hillard W, Koppes W, Linker D. Schwartz G. Digital signal and image processing in echocardiography. The American Society of Echocardiography. American Heart Journal.1985; 110:1266–1283.

3. Ten Cate FJ, Cornel JH, Serruys PW, Vletter WB, Roelandt J. Mittertreiner WH. Quantitative assessment of myocardial blood flow by contrast two-dimensional echocardiography: initial clinical observations. American Journal of Physiologic Imaging 1987; 2:56–60.

4. Kemper AJ, Force T, Kloner R, Gilfoil M, Perkins L, Hale S, Alker K, Parisi AF. Contrast echocardiographicestimation of regional myocardial blood flow after acute coronary occlusion. Circulation 1985; 72:1115–24.

5. Sklenar J, Jayaweera AR, Kaul S. A computer-aided approach for the quantitation of regional left ventricular function using two-dimensional echocardiography. J Am Soc Echocardiography 1992; 5:33–40.

6. Jayaweera AR, Skyba DM, Kaul S. Technical factors that influence the determination of microbubble transit rate during contrast echocardiography. J Am Soc Echocardiography 1995; 8:198–206.

7. Jayaweera AR, Matthew TL, Sklenar J, Spotnitz WD, Watson DD, Kaul S. Method for the quantitation of myocardial perfusion during myocardial contrast two-dimensional echocardiography. J Am Soc Echocardiography 1990; 3:91–98.

8. Jayaweera AR, Sklenar J, Kaul S. Quantification of images obtained during myocardial contrast echocardiography. Echocardiography 1994; 11:385–396.

9. Vandenberg BF, Kieso R, Fox-Eastham K, Chilian W, Kerber RE. Quantitation of myocardial perfusion by contrast echocardiography: analysis of contrast grey level appearance variables and intra-cyclic variability. J Am Coll Cardiol 1989; 13:200–206.

10. Jayaweera AR, Sklenar J, Kaul S. Quantification of images obtained during myocardial contrast echo-cardiography. Echocardiography 1994; 11:385–396.

11. Wei K, Skyba D M, Firschke C, Jayaweera AR, Lindner J R, Kaul S. Interactions between micro-bubbles and ultrasound: in vitro and in vivo observations. J Am Coll Cardiol 1997; 29:1081–1088.

12. Wei K, Jayaweera AR, Firoozan S, Linka A, Skyba DM, Kaul S. Quantification of myocardial blood flow with ultrasound-induced destruction of microbubbles administered as a continuous venous infusion. Circulation 1998; 97:473–483.

A Contrast Glossary

Aliasing
The situation that arises when the Nyquist sampling limit (one half of the PRF for pulsed Doppler systems) is exceeded by the frequency of the input signal.

Amplitude
The magnitude of a quantity such as frequency or of a wave variable such as velocity, displacement, or acceleration.

Amplitude map
A colour Doppler display in which the colours correspond to the amplitude of the Doppler signal, rather than to the Doppler shift frequency.

Array
A spatial arrangement of two or more transducers or transducer elements. An array may be linear (elements arranged along a line), curvilinear (elements arranged along a convex curve), rectangular (elements arranged in a rectangular pattern), annular (elements arranged in concentric circles).

Artifact
A feature of an image which does not correspond to reality. Reverberations and shadowing are examples of imaging artifacts; aliasing is an example of a Doppler artifact.

Attenuation
Decrease in the intensity of sound as it travels through a material. Three factors contribute to acoustic attenuation: absorption, scattering and beam divergence.

Autocorrelation
A mathematical procedure whereby a waveform is multiplied by successively time-shifted sections of itself. The autocorrelation method can be used to quantify periodicity in a Doppler signal and forms the basis of most colour Doppler velocity estimators.

Backscatter
The energy reradiated by a scatterer in a direction opposite to that of the incident wave.

Backscatter energy
The portion of the incident acoustic energy scattered back toward the source.

Bandwidth
The range of frequencies present in a signal. The bandwidth is defined as that portion of the signal's frequency spectrum between upper and lower frequency bounds.

Beam-vessel angle
The angle between the axis of the ultrasound beam and the axis of a vessel lumen. This will only be equal to the Doppler angle when flow is parallel to the vessel axis. Also known as angle of attack.

Bernoulli effect
The reduction in pressure that accompanies an increase in velocity of fluid flow.

Bernoulli equation
The equation which states that the total fluid energy along a streamline of fluid of flow is constant. This is a form of the more general law of conservation of energy.

Bernoulli, Daniel (1700–1782)
Swiss mathematician, sometimes referred to as the founder of mathematical physics, who unified the study of hydrodynamics under what became known later as the principle of the conservation of energy. Daniel Bernoulli was one of an extraordinary dynasty of eight mathematicians spanning three generations of the same family. Their collective contributions to mathematics and science are too numerous to list.

Bolus
In contrast imaging, a rapid injection of material. From the Greek for 'clump'.

Boundary layer
The thin layer of quasi-stationary fluid in contact with the walls of the containing vessel.

Bubble population
The ensemble of bubbles which comprise a contrast agent dose. Note that the distribution of such parameters as bubble radius and shell thickness changes once the agent has experienced transpulmonary passage.

Bubble specific imaging
Imaging method designed to suppress the echo from tissue in relation to that from a microbubble contrast agent.

Centre frequency
In a pulsed ultrasound system, the median frequency of the transmitted pulse. The pulse contains a range of frequencies.

Cineloop
A period of image, colour or spectral Doppler data stored digitally as a sequence of individual frames in system memory. A cineloop can be played at any speed, transferred to videotape or an archiving medium. Cineloops recorded at high frame rates will contain more frames than were displayed to the operator on the video display during the examination.

Clutter
Unwanted structural components of the received signal (for example, Doppler shifts from moving solid tissues). In contrast imaging, clutter often refers to the portion of the received echo that is not from microbubble contrast.

Coherence
The degree of phase agreement among the signals making up a composite wave; if all the signals are in phase, the wave is said to be coherent. There are various degrees of coherence that describe waves with less than full coherence. If no phase agreement exists the wave is called incoherent.

Colour Doppler imaging
A form of pulsed Doppler in which a large number of estimates of Doppler shift frequency are colour-coded and overlaid in the location of their detection on the greyscale image. Colour Doppler imaging systems operate within the range of 'real-time' frame rates. Also referred to as 'colour flow imaging'.

Glossary

Colour map
In a colour Doppler display, the allocation of colours to specific Doppler shift frequencies corresponding to flow in the forward and reverse directions. Colour maps may also be created to display Doppler signal power, amplitude, variance, or the grey levels of the B-mode image.

Colour priority
When both a B-mode echo and a Doppler shift is detected from the same location in a colour Doppler system, the colour-write priority determines which will be displayed in a given pixel. A low colour priority will allow solid tissue to conceal Doppler shifts at the same location, a high priority ensures that colour will overwrite the greyscale image. Also known as colour-echo write priority or angio write priority.

Compression
For a travelling acoustic wave, the rise in pressure of the medium during the positive portion of the acoustic cycle.

Contrast agent
A material which, when introduced into blood or tissue, causes one or more of its acoustic properties to change significantly. The most common of these properties is backscatter coefficient. Intravascular contrast agents usually comprise microbubbles which increase the blood echo level and can hence enhance the detectability of blood flow.

Conventional imaging
See Fundamental imaging

Correlation
For ultrasound, a mathematical procedure which is used to quantify the similarity between two signals.
Autocorrelation:
A mathematical procedure whereby a waveform is multiplied by successively time-shifted versions of itself. The autocorrelation method can be used to quantify periodicity or time variation in, for example, a Doppler signal.
Cross-correlation:
A mathematical procedure whereby one waveform is multiplied by successively time-shifted versions of another wave form. Cross-correlation of successive ultrasound echoes can be used to quantify movement of tissue, including blood.

Decibel (dB)
A unit which expresses the ratio of two numbers on a logarithmic scale. The dB 'difference' of the powers of two signals or waves is ten times the logarithm of their ratio; that of their amplitude is 20 times the logarithm of their ratio.

Densitometry
Measurement of the intensity of an area of an image from its grey levels. As ultrasound image grey levels generally bear a nonlinear relationship to echo amplitude, this technique is not suitable for quantitation or subtraction of contrast images.

Destruction-reperfusion
An indicator dilution method to measure flow which exploits the ability of ultrasound to disrupt a population of bubbles in a region of interest. Following their disruption, the rate at which the region is reoccupied by bubbles is used to deduce flowrate.
See Negative bolus.

Diastole
The relaxation period in the cardiac cycle in which the ventricles fill and the aortic and pulmonary valves are closed. Where visible in the velocity pulse, the dicrotic notch forms a convenient point marking the beginning of diastole.

Directional Doppler detection
Detection of Doppler signals in such a way that Doppler shifts due to targets approaching the transducer are distinguished from Doppler shifts due to targets moving away from the transducer. Directional detection is usually achieved by means of quadrature demodulation.

Doppler angle
The angle between the direction of movement of reflectors, such as red blood cells, and the effective direction of the ultrasonic beam, which is normal to the wavefront.

Doppler velocity signal
A signal whose instantaneous voltage is proportional to the instantaneous Doppler frequency shift, derived by a frequency-to-voltage conversion of the Doppler signal.

Doppler, Christian Andreas (1805–1853)
Son of an Austrian stonemason, Doppler became Professor of Mathematics in Prague. He enunciated his principle in 1842 but, unfortunately, confused its interpretation (he was, it turned out, incorrectly using it to attempt to explain the colour of binary starts). The acoustical Doppler effect was demonstrated in 1845 by Buys Ballot using a trumpeter riding on a steam locomotive, which was loaned for the occasion by the Dutch government.

Doppler, continuous wave
An ultrasonic system that detects Doppler-shifted signals by continuous and simultaneous transmission of sound and reception of echoes. The CW Doppler provides no range resolution.

Doppler, pulsed
A range-measuring ultrasonic system that detects Doppler-shifted signals by collecting samples, each sample taken from a separate ultrasonic pulse collected from the same location in space.

Duplex scanner
An ultrasound instrument that has real-time imaging capability with either the imaging transducer or a separate transducer used to collect continuous-wave or pulsed Doppler signals, either simultaneously with imaging or sequentially. Often used to refer to a device which combines a pulsed Doppler with a spectral display and a real time imaging system.

Dynamic range
The ratio of the largest discernible signal to the smallest detectable signal in a system. This is a measure of the domain of linear operation of the system. For a Doppler system it is usually equal to the ratio between the maximum clutter signal and the minimum detectable signal while both signals are present (the clutter-to-signal ratio).

Energy map
See power map.

Ensemble length
The number of pulses emitted by a colour Doppler imaging system to create a single line of Doppler data in the image. Also known as 'packet length'.

Far field (Frauenhofer zone)
The region of the ultrasound field in which the acoustic energy flow proceeds essentially as though coming from a point source located in the vicinity of the transducer. For an unfocused circular transducer assembly, the far field commonly is ascribed to ranges greater than S/l where S is the radiating cross-sectional area of the transducer and l is the acoustic wavelength in the medium.

Fast Fourier transform (FFT)
A numerical algorithm used to compute the frequency components present in a periodic function varying with, for example, time. The Doppler signal is an example of such a function; the FFT produces an estimate of the relative amplitude of each frequency components, known as the Doppler spectrum.

Filter
A device used for suppressing acoustic or electromagnetic waves of certain frequencies while allowing others to pass.

Filter, highpass
A device which allows high – but not low – frequency variations to pass through. An example is the electrical filter used in Doppler devices to eliminate low-frequency Doppler shifts caused by clutter. This is also referred to as the 'wall' or 'thump' filter.

Filter, lowpass
A device that allows low – but not high – frequency variations to pass through. An example is a stenosis, which has the effect of damping rapid variations in the pressure and flow waveforms.

Flow phantom
A type of test object comprising a fluid containing ultrasound scatterers which is pumped through a pipe.

Flow rate
The volume of fluid passing through a given vessel per unit time. Measured in milliliters per second or liters per minute.

Focus, transmit
The point on the axis of an ultrasonic beam where the width of the beam has a minimum value; generally, all the waves passing through the focus are in phase in relation to the surface of the transducer or to the electronic summing point of an electronically focused array. In contrast imaging, the focus is the point at which maximum bubble disruption can be expected to occur.

Focusing, dynamic
A method for controlling the axial position of the focus of an ultrasonic beam; often realised by phase control of the signals detected by a transducer array.

Fourier analysis
Mathematical technique for the representation of a periodic function (such as a time-varying waveform) as a sum of sinusoidal functions of different frequencies. Each of these constituent functions has a frequency that is an exact multiple of the same number. Fourier analysis allows the presentation of a Doppler signal in terms of the relative power of the various Doppler shift frequencies of which it is composed.

Fourier, Joseph (1768–1830)
Son of a French tailor who was persuaded to leave his Benedictine monastery to become a Professor of Mathematics at the age of 21. Among his many original and outstanding contributions to mathematical physics is the analytic theory of heat, which Lord Kelvin called "a great mathematical poem". Some say that his death was speeded by his insistence that heat was good for the health and his later habit of living in rooms "hotter than the Sahara desert".

Frame
A single ultrasound image.

Frame averaging
The addition of consecutive frames in real-time imaging to smooth temporal variation. A form of highpass filtering.

Frequency spectrum
The range of frequencies present in a signal recorded over some period of time.

Frequency, Doppler shift
The difference between the frequencies of the transmitted wave and of the echo received from a moving target.

Fundamental frequency
The natural or resonant frequency of a system. The first harmonic of a system's oscillation.

Fundamental imaging
Term used to describe imaging and Doppler modes in which the detected signal is acquired and processed under the assumption of linear propagation and scattering.

Harmonic
Oscillation of a system at a frequency that is a simple multiple of its fundamental frequency of sinusoidal motion. The fundamental frequency of a sinusoidal oscillation is usually called the first harmonic. The second harmonic has a frequency twice that of the fundamental, and so on.

Harmonic imaging
Ultrasound technique in which echoes at higher harmonics (usually the second) of the transmitted fundamental frequency are detected preferentially. These echoes may originate from nonlinear scatterers, such as microbubbles of a contrast agent, or from linear scattering of sound which has undergone nonlinear propagation and hence developed harmonics.

Harmonic power angio
See Harmonic power Doppler.

Harmonic power Doppler
A contrast specific imaging mode in which a power Doppler imaging is formed from echoes detected at the second harmonic of the transmitted frequency. Because power Doppler is sensitive to echoes which decorrelate with time, this method is most effective at detecting bubbles undergoing disruption. The harmonic filtering helps suppress linear tissue motion.

Hertz
The unit of frequency, defined as one cycle per second.

Hydrophone
A transducer designed for underwater measurement of acoustic fields. The diameter of a hydrophone should be smaller than the wavelength of ultrasound to be measured, and its bandwidth should be large.

Impedance, acoustic
The product of speed of sound and density of a medium in which sound is traveling. Changes in acoustic impedance are responsible for the echoes on which ultrasound imaging and Doppler flow detection are based.

Indicator dilution
Method for measuring flow in which a detectable tracer is injected in the flowstream and its rate of dispersal by transit in the flow system measured.

Infusion
A steady, usually slow injection of material. With contrast agents, often achieved by means of a pump.

Intensity
The intensity (I) of a wave is the rate of energy flux (power) through a unit area perpendicular to the direction of propagation. The unit of intensity is watts per square meter (W/cm^2). The definitions of intensity commonly used in diagnostic ultrasound are:

Pulse-average intensity
The instantaneous intensity at a point in space, averaged over the duration of a single pulse.

Spatial-average intensity
The same as the spatial-average temporal-average intensity. Generally, this parameter is used when specifying the intensity for continuous-wave (CW) ultrasound.

Spatial-average pulse-average intensity (SAPA)
The pulse average intensity averaged over the beam cross-sectional area.

Spatial-average temporal-average intensity (SATA)
The temporal average intensity averaged over the beam cross-sectional area in a specified plane.

Spatial-peak pulse-average intensity (SPPA)
The value of the pulse average intensity at the point in the acoustic field where the pulse average intensity is a maximum, or is a local maximum within a specified region.

Spatial-peak temporal-peak intensity (SPTP)
The value of temporal peak intensity at the point in the acoustic field where the temporal peak intensity is a maximum, or is a local maximum within a specified region.

Temporal-average intensity
The time-average of instantaneous intensity at a point in space; this is equal to the mean value of the instantaneous intensity at the point considered. For scanning systems, the instantaneous intensity is averaged over one or more scan repetition periods for a specified operating mode.

Temporal peak intensity
The peak value of the instantaneous intensity at the point considered. It is given by $\frac{P^2}{\rho c}$, where P is the instantaneous acoustic pressure, ρ is the density of the medium and c is the speed of sound in the medium.

Interference
The phenomenon describing the interaction between two waves of the same or different frequencies to produce a resultant wave, the amplitude of which depends on the amplitude and phase relationship of the interfering waves.

Kelvin, Lord (1824–1907)
British physicist and president of the Royal Society; exponent of the principle that heavier-than-air flying machines are impossible.

Laminar flow
Flow in which there is smooth and gradual variation of velocity with position and with time. Flow may be thought of as comprising a series of individual laminae, each moving at one velocity, with viscous cohesion maintaining the flow of adjacent laminae at nearly the same velocity.

Line density
The number of lines transmitted by the ultrasound transducer per imaging frame. In contrast imaging, low line density can reduce bubble destruction.

Linear imaging
See Fundamental imaging.

Linear phased array
Term used to refer to a linear switched array which, in Doppler mode, operates a subset of its elements as a linear phased array and can thus steer the Doppler beam at a selected angle to the imaging beam. A popular configuration for peripheral vascular scanning.

Loss of correlation imaging
A term sometimes applied misleadingly to describe conventional power or colour Doppler imaging when used to detect bubble disruption.

Mechanical Index
Part of the AIUM/NEMA Real Time Output Display Standard for the labelling of acoustic output on diagnostic ultrasound systems. It is defined as the peak rarefactional pressure (expressed in MPa) when a simple, uniform medium is scanned, divided by the square root of the centre frequency of the pulse. The medium is assumed to have an attenuation of 0.3 dB/cm-MHz. *See also* Thermal Index.

Microbubble
In contrast imaging, a gas bubble stabilised by a thin shell, usually smaller in diameter than a red blood cell.

Motion discrimination detector
A class of signal processing used in colour Doppler systems which attempts to distinguish between Doppler shifts from moving blood (which the system normally seeks to display) and Doppler shifts from moving tissue (which the system normally seeks to suppress). This processing is especially important when the velocities of moving tissue and blood are similar, such as in the detection of small vessel flow.

Multiple frame trigger
A trigger, usually from the ECG, that initiates the acquisition of a series of consecutive frames. Used in triggered harmonic power Doppler modes to identify motion artifact in perfusion imaging.

Native harmonic imaging
See Tissue harmonic imaging.

Near field (Fresnel zone)
The region closest to the transducer. In contrast to the far field, the near field is characterised by inhomogeneity in acoustic pressure. For an unfocused circular transducer assembly, the near field commonly is ascribed to ranges less than S/l where S is the radiating cross-sectional area of the transducer and l is the acoustic wavelength in the medium.

Negative bolus
Term used to describe the exploitation of ultrasound's ability to destroy steadily infused microbubbles at a specific location in the circulation, thus creating a bolus defined by the absence of bubbles, which can be used as an indicator. *See* Destruction-reperfusion.

Noise
Random, and usually unwanted, signals.

Noise, electrical
Noise signals arising within the electrical circuits.

Nonlinear imaging
Ultrasound imaging designed to protect preferentially nonlinear components of the received echo. Harmonic and pulse inversion imaging are examples of nonlinear imaging methods.

Nonlinear propagation
The distortion of a wavefront propagating in a medium in which the compressional phase moves slightly faster than the rarefactional phase. The result is the conversion of some of the wave energy into higher harmonics of the fundamental frequency. The effect increases strongly with increasing wave amplitude.

Nonlinear scattering
The formation of an echo from a target undergoing oscillation with components at higher harmonics. In the case of a microbubble in an acoustic field, the oscillation is asymmetric with time, producing echoes with even harmonics.

Nyquist criterion
The criterion that a continuously varying signal can only be unambiguously represented by instantaneous samples if the sampling rate is more than twice the maximum frequency present in the signal.

Nyquist limit
The highest frequency in a sampled signal that can be represented unambiguously; equal to one-half of the sampling frequency. In Doppler systems, this is one-half of the repetition rate for flows in each direction.

Opacification
In contrast studies, the filling of an echo-free area, such as a ventricular cavity, with echoes from microbubble contrast.

Perfluorocarbons
Compounds obtained by replacing the hydrogen atoms of hydrocarbons by fluorine atoms. Their stability, inertness, low solubility and low diffusion constant make them suitable gases for microbubble contrast agents.

Perfusion imaging
Imaging of flow or blood volume at the capillary level. Because the flow velocities are comparable or lower than tissue velocities, conventional Doppler methods will not suffice.

Persistence
A form of temporal smoothing used in both greyscale and colour Doppler imaging in which successive frames are averaged as they are displayed. The effect is to reduce the variations in the image between frames, hence lowering the temporal resolution of the image. *See* Frame averaging.

Phantom
A device which simulates some parameters of the human body, allowing measurements of ultrasound system parameters or visualisation of simulated anatomical features.

Phantom, Doppler
A phantom designed to provide an acoustic simulation of biological tissue containing moving scatterers, usually blood.

Phase inversion imaging
See Pulse inversion imaging.

Phase quadrature
A signal-processing technique depending on an input signal being available both with its original phase and shifted through 90° of phase angle.

Phase, angle of
The numerical value of the angle of rotation of the vector describing a periodic wave; waves that are in phase have simultaneously occurring maxima (and zero crossings and minima); the maximum of a wave that is in antiphase with another wave occurs at the same time as the minimum of the other wave.

Phased array
A transducer configuration which consists of several piezoelectric elements which can be excited independently. Using proper time delays of the excitations, a wavefront of the desired configuration can be synthesised. Phased arrays have been utilised for electronic beam steering and focusing.

Poiseuille, Jean Leonard M. (1797–1869)
French physician and physicist who performed the first experiments demonstrating viscosity in a fluid and its relationship to pressure gradient in a tube. Poiseuille also refined the techniques of Hales for measuring pressure in the arterial circulation.

Poiseuille's law
Law stating that the fluid resistance in a long, straight tube with steady, irrotational flow is proportional to its length and viscosity and inversely proportional to the fourth power of its radius.

Power
The energy delivered by a wave or in a signal per unit of time; measured in watts (W).

Glossary

Power mode
A colour Doppler display in which the colours correspond to the power of the Doppler signal, rather than to its frequency.

Power pulse inversion
See Pulse inversion Doppler.

Power spectrum
A graph showing the relative power of each frequency component in a periodic function. For a Doppler signal, the power spectrum gives the distribution of Doppler shift frequencies present in the signal.

Pressure
A form of potential energy in a fluid. Pressure is defined as the force acting on each square meter of an imaginary plane facing any direction in a fluid.

Pressure, peak
The maximum pressure of the fluid medium (for eg. tissue) obtained during propagation of an ultrasound pulse.

Pressure, peak negative
The peak rarefaction pressure obtained during the negative portion of a propagating ultrasound pulse in a medium such as tissue.

Pressure, peak rarefactional
See Pressure, peak negative.

Pulse inversion Doppler
Nonlinear imaging method in which a sequence of pulses is transmitted into tissue whose phase or amplitude is changed from pulse to pulse in an incremental way. The received echoes are detected using fundamental or harmonic Doppler processing. The result is a Doppler spectrum whose Doppler shift frequencies reflect not only target velocity, but whether the target echoes are linear or nonlinear. This method forms the basis of the separation of microbubble echoes at low mechanical index, allowing real-time perfusion imaging.

Pulse inversion imaging
Nonlinear imaging method whereby two pulses are transmitted into tissue, the second an inverted copy of the first. The received echoes are summed, cancelling echoes from linear structures and enhancing echoes with even harmonic components.

Pulse Repetition Frequency (PRF)
The repetition of the transmission pulses of a pulse-echo system; the inverse of the pulse repetition period. Typically, the PRF of a system is in the range of 1 kHz to 20 kHz.

Range gate
An electronic circuit for selecting an ultrasonic signal according to its depth along the ultrasonic beam by gating the signal with an appropriate time delay.

Range, dynamic
See Dynamic range.

Rarefaction
For a travelling acoustic wave, the reduction in pressure of the medium during the negative portion of the acoustic cycle.

Rayleigh Scattering
The name given to the deflection of waves by an ensemble of targets much smaller than the wavelength of the incident radiation. Red blood cells are Rayleigh scatterers to ultrasound. The intensity of ultrasound scattered back to the transducer by the Rayleigh process is proportional to the fourth power of frequency.

Rayleigh, Lord (1842–1919)
Born John William Strutt in Essex, England, third baron Rayleigh was the son of a Duke and member of Parliament for Essex. Although educated at Cambridge, where he became Cavendish Professor of Physics and eventually Chancellor, he carried out much of his work in his private laboratory at his home in Terling. He received the Nobel Prize for physics in 1904 for his experimental work on the atmospheric elements but is perhaps remembered better for his classic and comprehensive treatise on the theory of sound published in 1877.

Real-time
The acquisition and display of ultrasonic images at a sufficiently rapid rate that moving structure can be "seen" to move at their natural rate. Frame rates of about 15 frames per second or greater are considered real-time.

Receive gain
The amplification to which a detected echo is subjected by an ultrasound system. In nonlinear imaging, it is important to distinguish the effect of this from change in the transmit power.

Reflection
Change in the direction of propagation of a wave as it encounters an interface between two media across which the acoustic impedance changes. The amplitude of the reflected wave is determined by the magnitude of this difference.

Reflection, specular
The phenomenon of reflection of a wave by a flat surface large in relation to the wavelength.

Refraction
Change in the direction of propagation of a wave as it crosses an interface between two media with different speeds of sound. The amount by which the portion of the wave entering the second medium is deviated depends on the difference in propagation velocity between the media and the angle of incidence at their interface.

Resolution (spatial)
A measure of the ability of a system to display distinguishable images of two closely spaced point structures as discrete targets.

Resolution (temporal)
A measure of the ability of a system to display two closely spaced events in time as discrete entities.

Resonance
Oscillation of a system at its natural frequency of vibration, as determined by the physical parameters of the system. At resonance, large amplitude vibrations will ultimately result from low-power driving of the system. Resonance can occur in microbubbles driven by an acoustic wave. The resonant frequency for a free gas bubble is primarily determined by its size.

Reynolds Number
A number expressing the balance of inertial and viscous forces acting on a flowing fluid. Reynolds numbers higher than a critical value result in disturbed flow progressing to turbulent flow.

Reynolds stress
The increased resistance to flow offered by a fluid in turbulence, which has its origin in viscous forces resulting from chaotically oriented velocity gradients.

Reynolds, Sir Osborne (1842–1912)
English mechanical and civil engineer who pioneered the study of vortical and turbulent flow in liquids and laid the theoretical basis for subsequent study of the behaviour of viscous fluids. Reynolds also built a steam engine for the determination of mechanical equivalent of heat and held patents for the design of marine turbines.

Sample volume
The region of the ultrasound beam (or beams in a CW system) sensitive to the presence of Doppler-shifted echoes. In a pulsed Doppler system, the axial position and extent of the sample volume is determined by the length of the transmitted pulse and the location and length of the range gate, both of which are normally under control of the operator. The sample volume width is determined by the lateral extent of the ultrasound beam.

Scatterer
A discontinuity small in relation to the wavelength that reradiates ultrasound through an angle rather than in specular fashion.

Shell
For a microbubble, the coating which stablises the gas contents of a microbubble within the fluid medium. In ultrasound contrast agents, the shell is made from a lipid, protein, or other biocompatible material.

Sideband
The components of a signal whose frequencies are either above (upper sideband) or below (lower sideband) the frequency of the (carrier) transmitted signal.

Signal-noise ratio (SNR)
The ratio of the amplitude of a signal to that of noise. The larger the signal-noise ratio, the easier it is to detect and measure a signal. The sensitivity of any device is ultimately limited by the signal-noise ratio. The SNR is usually expressed in decibels.

Signal-to-Clutter Ratio (SCR)
The ratio of the amplitude of the wanted portion of a Doppler signal to that of its largest clutter component. The larger the signal-clutter ratio, the easier it is to distinguish Doppler shifts due to blood flow from those of other targets. Because the clutter is usually much greater in amplitude than the wanted signal in clinical Doppler examinations, the SCR is a primary determinant of the detectability of flow in a given vessel. It is usually expressed in decibels.

Sound
Vibrational energy that propagates through a medium. Liquids and gases support longitudinal (compression) waves. Solids support other vibration modes in addition to longitudinal waves.

Spectral broadening
The width of the Doppler spectrum on a sonogram display, which corresponds to the range of Doppler shift frequencies present at a given time. Spectral broadening will be seen to increase when this range is increased; one example is the Doppler signal obtained when laminar flow with a blunt flow profile becomes disturbed.

Spectral Doppler
A name commonly used to refer to the combination of either CW or pulsed Doppler with a spectral display.

Spectral width
Estimate of range of frequencies present in a spectrum, defined as the difference between the upper bandwidth frequency and lower bandwidth frequency.

Spectrum
A range of values, often continuous; for example, the range of frequencies in a Doppler-shifted signal.

Stimulated acoustic emission
A term sometimes used to refer to transient echoes from bubbles undergoing disruption.

Subharmonic
An oscillation of a system at a frequency that is a simple fraction of that of its fundamental sinusoidal oscillation. The second subharmonic has a frequency of one half the fundamental frequency, and so on.

Systole
The pumping portion of the cardiac cycle during which the aortic valve is open. Identifiable from the Doppler waveform as the period from the foot of the velocity pulse to the dicrotic notch.

Target
A reflector, scatterer, or ensemble of scatterers giving rise to a detectable signal when within the effective ultrasonic beam.

Test object, Doppler
A device designed to create a reproducible acoustic and physical setting in which one or more aspects of a Doppler system's performance may be tested or calibrated.

Thermal Index
Part of the AIUM/NEMA Real Time Output Display Standard for the labelling of acoustic output on diagnostic ultrasound systems. It is defined as the ratio of the power being emitted to the power required to raise the temperature by 1 degree Celsius in a simple, uniform medium insonified by the active transducer. The medium is assumed to have an attenuation of 0.3 dB/cm-MHz. *See also* Mechanical Index.

Tissue harmonic imaging
Nonlinear imaging mode which preferentially detects echoes from higher harmonics of the fundamental transmitted signal, developed as a consequence of nonlinear propagation in tissue.

Transient echo
In contrast imaging, an echo of high intensity and short duration associated with disruption of a bubble, following its exposure to an acoustic field.

Glossary

Transit time broadening
The spectral broadening that occurs as a consequence of the movement of scatterers through a Doppler sample volume of finite size. The smaller the sample volume, the more pronounced is the transit time broadening. Also known as geometric or intrinsic spectral broadening.

Transmit intensity
The intensity of the pulse of sound emitted by the transducer into the body. For contrast imaging, the peak rarefactional pressure is a major determinant of bubble response.

Transmit power
Common name given to the control on an ultrasound system that determines transmit intensity. The total energy transmitted into tissue by the transducer.

Triggered imaging
The control of the acquisition of a single or series of ultrasound images by an external signal. In echocardiography the trigger is usually derived from the ECG signal.

Turbulence
Disorganised flow with chaotically oriented components in many directions. Occurs in disturbed flow when a critical value of the Reynolds number is exceeded.

Ultraharmonic
Oscillation of a system at a frequency that is a rational multiple of that of its fundamental sinusoidal oscillation, for example 1.5 or 2.5 times the fundamental frequency.

Variance map
A colour Doppler display in which the saturation of a colour corresponds to the estimated variance of the Doppler signal. This is often combined with the velocity map by using a different hue, so that the combination of the two quantities can be used for the detection of turbulence.

Vector
Quantity defined with both the magnitude and the direction. Velocity is a vector quantity; the Doppler shift frequency is determined by the magnitude of the component of the velocity vector along a line between the source and the receiver of sound.

Velocity
A vector describing the rate of change of position with time. Also used for the magnitude of the velocity vector, although this quantity is really the flow 'speed'.

Velocity gradient
The rate of change of velocity with position. With steady laminar flow in a round vessel, this gradient is usually in a radial direction.

Velocity profile
The variation of velocity with radial position for flow in a vessel.

Velocity profile, blunted
A modification of the parabolic flow profile that is commonly encountered in physiological circumstances. The central laminae move at almost one velocity.

Velocity profile, parabolic
The form of the velocity profile found with steady flow in a round vessel that exhibits flow resistance only. The parabolic flow profile has the special property that the average velocity across the vessel is exactly one-half of the maximum velocity in the centre stream. Also called Poiseuille flow.

Velocity, critical
The flow velocity at which the Reynolds number attains its critical value and the transition of disturbed flow to turbulence occurs.

Wall filter
A highpass filter designed to exclude low frequency, high amplitude Doppler signals from moving solid tissue, such as a vessel wall. Wall filter performance is critical to the success of a colour Doppler system.

Wall thump
A strong, low-frequency clutter signal tending to obscure the Doppler frequency spectrum of interest, often arising from motion of the walls of a blood vessel.

Index

A

Acoustic window, for myocardial perfusion imaging 88
Acute myocardial infarction
–, interpretation of perfusion images 121–123
–, need for imaging 83–84
Acute transmural infarction, indication for contrast echo 86
Adenosine stress
–, during myocardial perfusion imaging 109–111
–, for coronary flow reserve 137
–, protocol for coronary flow reserve 138
Albunex 6
Aliasing 25
–, defined 172
Alignment
–, automatic 158–159
–, of images offline 157–159
American Society of Echocardiography
–, myocardial segment model 51, 112, 156
Amplitude
–, defined 172
–, map 25, see also Power mode
Angio priority, for perfusion imaging 105
Anti-contrast
–, artifact 63, 67
Artifact
–, defined 172
–, anti-contrast 63, 67
–, attenuation 57
–, attenuation in perfusion imaging 129–130
–, blooming in perfusion imaging 131
–, bubble depletion 133
–, bubble noise 145
–, colour blooming 76
Doppler angle 143
–, in LV opacification, avoiding 77
–, myocardial contrast as 75
–, near field 66
–, reverberation 29
–, sample volume displacement 144
–, sidelobe 29
–, wall motion 74
–, wall motion in myocardial perfusion imaging 131–132
Attenuation 62, 66
–, and conventional imaging 19
–, defined 172
Automatic image alignment 158–159

B

Background subtraction 91
Backscatter, defined 172
Bandwidth
–, and harmonic imaging 29–31
–, defined 172
–, transducer 23
Before you inject 55
Bernoulli effect, defined 172
Bifurcation rate 3
Bioeffects, potential for 40–41
Blood pool agents 5
Blood pressure, impact on coronary flow reserve measurement 146
Blooming, in myocardial perfusion imaging 131
B-mode gain, for perfusion imaging 104
B-mode imaging
–, conventional 2
–, for coronary flow reserve 140
B-mode imaging for LV opacification 56–58
Bolus
–, defined 172
–, pros and cons 14
–, time behaviour 156
–, time course 12
–, versus infusion 14–16
Bolus injection, time course 164
Bubble depletion artifact, in myocardial perfusion imaging 133
Bubble disruption artifact 64, 67
Bubble noise, in coronary flow reserve studies 145
Bubble population, defined 172
Bubble specific imaging 20–24
–, defined 172

C

Canadian consensus recommendations, for diastolic dysfunction 61
Capillary flow 82–84
Cavitation 40–41
Cineloop
–, defined 172
–, processing 159–164
Clutter 20
–, defined 172
Coded harmonic angio 104
Colour blooming, artifact 76
Colour box, size/position 104
Colour Doppler
–, for LV opacification 70
–, role in pulmonary venous measurement 61
Colour Doppler imaging
–, defined 172
–, for coronary flow reserve 140
Colour gain
–, adjusting 102
–, for perfusion imaging 104
Colour power angio 104
Colour power angiography 25, See also Harmonic power Doppler
Colour priority
–, defined 172
–, for perfusion imaging 105
Colour threshold 102
–, for perfusion imaging 105
Continuous imaging, for LV opacification 68
Contraindications, for perfusion echo 88
Contrast agent
–, administration of 12
–, blood pool 6
–, defined 173
–, dose-response 13
–, encapsulated air 6
–, encapsulated perfluorocarbon 7
–, free gas 6
–, ideal 5
–, infusion of 99-100
–, injection of 11
–, need for 2
–, types 5–8
–, evolution of 8
–, for therapy 41–42
–, preparation of 10
–, selective uptake 8

Index   181

–, storage of 10
–, tissue specific 41
Contrast for LV opacification
–, B-mode 56
–, indications 51
–, instrument settings 56
Contrast for PV Doppler, indications 53
Conventional imaging
–, defined 173
–, for PV Doppler 53–55
Coronary angiography, in LAD stenosis 137
Coronary artery stenosis
–, perfusion defects 124–127
–, as indication for perfusion imaging 86–87
Coronary flow reserve 85, 133–147
–, and myocardial contrast echo 87–88
–, clinical methods available 136
–, combination with myocardial perfusion imaging 141
–, defined 134
–, for LAD stenosis 143
–, image acquisition 142–143
–, image interpretation 143–144
–, in the 'difficult' patient 137
–, indications 135–137
–, pitfalls 143–144
–, selection of patients 136
–, and blood pressure 146
–, and preload 146

D

Data reduction, using offline software 156
Decibel, defined 173
Definity 8
Densitometry, defined 173
Destruction frame, for quantitation of real-time perfusion imaging 168–170
Destruction-reperfusion 165–167
–, defined 173
–, *See also* Negative bolus technique
Diastole, defined 173
Diastolic function 50–51, 48–49
DICOM network 108
Dilution, of contrast agent 15
Dipyridamole stress
–, during myocardial perfusion imaging 109–111
–, for coronary flow reserve 137
–, protocol for coronary flow reserve 138
Dobutamine stress, during myocardial perfusion imaging 109
Doppler
–, continuous wave, defined 173
–, conventional 3
–, detection threshold 3
–, performance limits 4
–, pulsed, defined 173
–, small vessel 4
–, intracoronary 134
Doppler angle
–, defined 173
–, in coronary flow reserve studies 143
Doppler enhancement 18–20
Doppler scale, explained 104
Doppler sensitivity 105, *See also* Ensemble length, Packet length
Dose, contrast agent
–, for LV opacification 57–58
–, for myocardial perfusion imaging 100

–, for pulmonary venous Doppler 61
–, harmonic imaging for LV opacification 63
–, harmonic power Doppler for LV opacification 70
–, triggered Doppler imaging for LV opacification 74
Drug delivery, with contrast agents 41–42
Dual display 104
Duplex Doppler 2
–, defined 173
Duration of enhancement 13
Dynamic range 105
–, defined 173

E

Echovist 7
Echogen 7
Ejection fraction 48
–, how to measure with contrast echo 72–74
–, triggered imaging for 72
Endocardial border
–, definition 51
–, visualisation score 51
Energy map, defined 174
Enhancement
–, duration 13
–, integrated fractional 14
–, peak 13
Ensemble length 105
–, defined 173
Exercise stress, during myocardial perfusion imaging 109
Exponential function, for quantitative perfusion measurement 165–170

F

Fast Fourier transform, defined 174
False defect, in myocardial perfusion imaging 130
Filter, defined 174
Fixed defects, on myocardial perfusion imaging 116
Flash artifact 5
Flash echo
–, for perfusion imaging 95–96
–, for quantitation of real-time perfusion 169–170
–, real-time with power pulse inversion 96–97
Flowrate, defined 174
Flush, saline 11–12
Focus, transmit 104
–, defined 174
Fourier analysis, defined 174
Fragmentation, microbubble 36
Frame
–, defined 174
–, for myocardial perfusion imaging 104
Frame averaging
–, defined 174
–, for perfusion imaging 105
Frame-rate
–, for perfusion imaging 105
–, in pulse inversion imaging 31
Frequency
–, Doppler shift, defined 174
–, Fundamental, defined 174

G

Galactose particles, for contrast 6
Gamma variate model, in offline analysis 165
Global LV function 49–50

H

Harmonic, defined 174
Harmonic power Doppler 25
Harmonic colour Doppler imaging 68, *See also* Harmonic power Doppler imaging
Harmonic Doppler, quantitative performance 27
Harmonic emission, from microbubble contrast agent 22
Harmonic imaging
–, defined 174
–, B-mode 23
–, B-mode, perfusion settings 103
–, Doppler 23–25
–, extension of image lifetime 27
–, for LV opacification 63–67
–, for perfusion imaging 90–91
–, impact of 26–27
–, limitations 30
–, of LV thrombi 67–68
–, of tissue 28, *See also* Tissue harmonic imaging
Harmonic imaging modalities, summary of 28
Harmonic power Doppler
–, defined 174
–, for ejection fraction 55
–, for LV opacification 68–77
–, pitfalls in LV opacification 72
–, settings for LV opacification 71
–, settings for myocardial perfusion imaging 100–102
–, for myocardial perfusion imaging 89–90
Harmonic power Doppler imaging 25
Harmonic response, of microbubble 21
Harmonic spectral Doppler, for clutter suppression 24
Hemolysis 41
High pass filter, and Doppler detection 4, *See also* Wall filter
Histogram display, of contrast effect 155–158
Hyperemea, with vasodilation 147

I

Image acquisition
–, for coronary flow reserve 142–143
–, for LV opacification 63–64
–, for perfusion imaging 109–110
–, for pulmonary venous Doppler 61–62
Image alignment 157–159
Image processing, for myocardial contrast echo 154–158
Image quantification, basic tools 154–156
Inadequate myocardial contrast, in perfusion studies 127–128
Indicator dilution
–, and negative bolus method 166–167
–, defined 175
Infusion
–, defined 175
–, for perfusion imaging 97–99
–, necessity for 14–16
Infusion versus bolus, for perfusion imaging 97–99
Instrument settings for
–, coronary flow reserve using Doppler imaging 140
–, coronary flow reserve using spectral Doppler 141
–, LV opacification using B-mode 56
–, LV opacification using harmonic Doppler 71
–, LV opacification using real-time harmonic B-mode 64
–, LV opacification using triggered harmonic power Doppler 73
–, myocardial perfusion 100–108
–, myocardial perfusion using harmonic B-mode 103
–, myocardial perfusion using harmonic power Doppler 102
–, myocardial perfusion using pulse inversion 106
–, myocardial perfusion using real-time power pulse inversion 107
–, pulmonary venous Doppler 59–60
–, understanding perfusion imaging settings 104–105
Integrated fractional enhancement 14
Intensity, defined 175
Intermittent harmonic power Doppler, principles 37–39
Intermittent imaging
–, explained 36–38
–, for myocardial perfusion 94–97, *See also* Triggered imaging
Interpretation, of myocardial perfusion imaging studies, 121–125
Interpretation of myocardial contrast images, clinical profiles 121–128
Intravital microscopy, of microbubble agent 8
Ischemic cascade 85
Ischemic heart disease, chronic 83–84

K

Kupffer cells 8

L

LAD stenosis
–, assessment with coronary flow reserve 143
–, follow-up after PTCA 143
Lateral wall, dropout 115–116
Left anterior descending coronary artery 135–136, 139
Left ventricular function
–, methods of assessment 49
–, physiology and pathophysiology 48–51
–, role of contrast 49
Left ventricular thrombi 52
Left ventricular function, selection of imaging methods 54–56
Levovist 6
Line density
–, defined 175
–, in perfusion imaging 105
Linear backscatter 18–20
Linear imaging, defined 175
Linear echo, cancellation 31
Logarithmic mapping, impact on subtraction 161
Loss of correlation imaging, defined 175
Low velocity reject, for perfusion imaging 105, *See also* Wall filter

M

Magneto-optical disks 108
Manual injection, of contrast agent 15
Mean velocity 166
Mechanical Index
–, and microbubble response 16–18
–, defined 175
–, explained 18
–, for myocardial perfusion imaging 89
Memory artery, artifact in coronary flow reserve studies, 144–145
MI, *See* Mechanical Index
Microbubble
–, acoustic response of 16
–, behaviour with incident pressure 17
–, concentration 154
–, defined 175
–, diffusion of gas from 38
–, disruption 36–38
–, fragmentation 36
–, effect of shell on resonance 22–23
–, encapsulated 6
–, free gas 6
–, mode of action 16
–, oscillation in an acoustic field 16–21
–, scattering from 16–24

Index

–, shell 7
–, shell, defined 178
–, tissue specific 41
Microvascular integrity 83
Multiple frame trigger, defined 175
Myocardial blood flow 83
Myocardial blood volume 83
Myocardial contrast, as artifact 75
Myocardial contrast echo
–, indications 86–88
–, why? 86
Myocardial perfusion
–, normal 82–83
–, physiology and pathophysiology of 82–84
Myocardial perfusion imaging
–, available methods 39
–, available ultrasound methods 88
–, combined with stress and wall motion studies 111–112
–, contraindications 88
–, normal perfusion 112–116
–, perfusion defect 116–119
–, reading studies 112–121
–, reducing artifacts 101–102
–, understanding instrument settings 104–105
Myocardial scintigraphy 85–86
Myocellular viability 86
Myocyte necrosis 83

N

Negative bolus
–, clinical technique 167–168
–, defined 176
Negative bolus technique 165–170
–, in real-time 169–170
–, principles 165–167
No reflow 87
Noise floor, impact on subtraction 161
–, defined 176
Nonlinear backscatter 20–24
Nonlinear imaging 20–24
–, defined 176
Nonlinear scattering, defined 176
Normal perfusion, visual assessment 113–116

O

Offline analysis 154
Opacification defined 176
Optison 7
Output power 104
Overtones 22, See also Harmonics

P

Parametric images, produced offline 169
Peak enhancement 13
Peak pressure, and microbubble response 17
Perfluorocarbons, defined 176
Perfusion defect
–, calling 118
–, due to coronary artery stenosis 124–127
–, when is it real? 121
Perfusion imaging
–, defined 176
–, summary of methods 39
–, understanding instrument settings 104–105
Perfusion rate 154, 166
Persistence 105

–, defined 176
Phase inversion imaging, See Pulse inversion imaging
Phase, angle of 176
Pick, in image analysis 155
Pitfalls
–, in coronary flow reserve studies 143–144
–, in harmonic imaging for LV opacification 63–64
–, in LV opacification studies 58
–, in myocardial perfusion imaging 127–133
–, in pulmonary venous Doppler 61–62
–, in triggered Doppler imaging for LVO 74–77
Positron emission tomography, for coronary flow reserve 136
Post processed recordings, visual assessment of 119–121
Post processing, of myocardial perfusion images 158–165
Power mode, defined 177
Power pulse inversion imaging
–, defined 177
–, flash echo 96–97
–, for myocardial perfusion 91–92
–, instrument settings for real-time perfusion 107–108
–, principles 34–36
–, real-time quantitative analysis 169–170
–, tissue suppression 35
Preload, impact on coronary flow reserve measurement 146
Pressure, peak acoustic 17
–, defined 177
Propagation velocity, and tissue harmonics 28
Pulmonary venous Doppler 59–63
–, indications for contrast 53
Pulmonary venous flow, and diastolic function 50–51
Pulse inversion, for myocardial perfusion imaging 91
Pulse inversion Doppler 34–36
–, defined 177, See also Power pulse inversion imaging
Pulse inversion imaging 31–33
–, defined 177
–, effect of low MI 33
–, for LV thrombi 68
–, principles 29–32
–, settings for perfusion 106
–, suppression of linear echoes 32
Pulse repetition frequency (PRF) 25, 102, 104
–, defined 177
–, in harmonic power Doppler 38
Pulsed wave Doppler, for pulmonary venous flow 59–63

Q

Quantification
–, of cineloop images 156–159
–, of single images 155–156

R

Rayleigh
–, law 20
–, Lord, bubbles and tea kettle 21, 177
–, scattering, defined 177
Real-time imaging
–, defined 177
–, for LV opacification 68–71
Real-time perfusion imaging 35, 91, 107
–, real-time quantitative negative bolus technique 169–170
Receive gain 65
–, defined 177
Region of interest
–, in offline analysis 155
–, positioning 156
Regional LV function 49–50

Report form
–, for perfusion stress imaging 127
–, for visual assessment of myocardial perfusion imaging 122
Reporting, visually assessed myocardial perfusion studies 121
Resolution
–, and harmonic imaging 29–31
–, defined 177
Resonance, microbubble 20–23
–, defined 177
Reverberation artifact 2, 29
Reversible defects, on myocardial perfusion imaging 116–118

S

Safety considerations 40–41
Saline flush 11–12
Sample volume
–, defined 178
–, displacement 62–63
–, displacement in coronary flow reserve studies 144
Scale, in the vascular system 82
Scatterer, defined 178
Scanplane, for myocardial perfusion imaging 92–94
Scar or fibrosis, versus viable myocardium 123
Shadowing, in perfusion imaging 129–130
Shell
–, defined 178
–, microbubble 7
–, polymer 41
Sidelobe artifact 29
Signal-to-noise ratio, defined 178
Signal-to-clutter ratio, defined 178
Sololuminescence 40
Sonazoid 8, 9, 163
SonoVue 8, 9
Sound propagation 16
SPECT, for coronary flow reserve 137
Spectral blooming 61
Spectral Doppler
–, defined 178
–, for coronary flow reserve 141
Steal phenomenon, during vasodilator stress 109–110
Stress ECG 84
Stress echocardiography 51–52
–, for wall motion 84–85
Stress testing
–, combined perfusion and wall motion studies 111–112
–, during myocardial contrast echo 109–111
–, protocol with perfusion imaging 109
Subharmonic emission, from contrast agent 22
–, defined 178
Subtraction
–, pulse to pulse 37–38
–, background 160–164
Swirling 64
Systole, defined 178
Systolic function, need for contrast 49

T

Thallium imaging 86
Thermal index, defined 178
Thrombi, left ventricular 67–68
Time enhancement curves 12
Tissue echo, as an obstacle to perfusion imaging 93
Tissue harmonic imaging 28–29
–, defined 178
–, for LV opacification 50

–, with pulse inversion 32–34
Transducer
–, bandwidth 23
–, positioning for myocardial perfusion imaging 93
–, frequency 104
Transesophageal echocardiography 49
–, Doppler 134
Transient echo
–, defined 178
–, from microbubble disruption 36–39
Transient imaging 36–39, *See also* Intermittent/Triggered imaging
Transmit power
–, and LV opacification 65
–, defined 179
–, impact on LV opacification 67
Transmural gradient, of perfusion 84
Transmural steal phenomenon 83–84
Trigger
–, defined 179
–, position 104
–, systolic versus diastolic 97
Trigger intervals, in myocardial perfusion imaging 132–133
Trigger point, setting 101–102
Triggered imaging
–, double or multiple 95,
–, defined 179
–, explained 36–37
–, flash echo 95–96
–, for injection fraction 72–74
–, for LV opacification 72–74
–, for myocardial perfusion imaging 94–97
–, incremental 95
T-wave, setting for perfusion imaging 106

U

Ultraharmonic, defined 179
Unresolved flow 3

V

Variance map, defined 179
Vascular volume 154, 166
Vasodilator stress
–, during myocardial perfusion imaging 109–111
–, and hyperemea 147
Velocity gradient, defined 179
Velocity profile, defined 179
Viable myocardium, versus scar or fibrosis 123
Videotape 108
Visual assessment
–, of post processed recordings 119–121
–, of myocardial perfusion imaging, criteria 119

W

Wall filter 4, 105
–, defined 179
–, setting 102
Wall motion
–, assessment with contrast 68–71, *See also* Left ventricular opacification
–, for coronary artery disease 85
–, real-time studies with perfusion imaging 111–112
Wall motion artifact 74
–, in LV opacification studies 70
–, in myocardial perfusion imaging 131–132